Dyslexia

Other books by Dr. Robert E. Valett

The Remediation of Learning Disabilities
Programming Learning Disabilities
Modifying Children's Behavior
Prescriptions for Learning
Effective Teaching
Learning Disabilities: Diagnostic-Prescriptive Instruments
The Psychoeducational Treatment of Hyperactive Children
Affective-Humanistic Education
The Practice of School Psychology
Getting It All Together
The Valett Perceptual-Motor Transitions to Reading Program
Self-Actualization
Humanistic Education: Developing the Total Person
Developing Cognitive Abilities: Teaching Children to Think

Dyslexia

A Neuropsychological Approach to Educating Children with Severe Reading Disorders

Robert E. Valett, Ed.D.
California State University, Fresno

Fearon Education
a division of
PITMAN LEARNING, INC.
Belmont, California

To Aleksandr Romanovich Luria

who enabled me to think more carefully
about learning, cognition, and remedial education.

Acknowledgments Appreciation is extended to the following publishers for permission to reprint material in this book:

Page 22: Figure 32 from *The Working Brain: An Introduction to Neuropsychology* by A. R. Luria, © Penguin Books Ltd., 1973, translation © Penguin Books Ltd., 1973, Basic Books, Inc., Publishers, New York.

Page 178: "Learning the *M* Sound" from *Perceptual-Motor Transitions to Reading* by Robert Valett and Shirley Valett (San Rafael, Calif.: Academic Therapy Publications, 1974), pp. 43-47.

Pages 86 and 217: "Individual Profile of Learning Skills and Abilities" and "Cognitive Skills Instructional Taxonomy" from *Developing Cognitive Abilities—Teaching Children to Think* (St. Louis: The C. V. Mosby Co., 1978) pp. 188-89 and p. 50.

Page 234: "Dolch Basic Sight Vocabulary" by E. W. Dolch. Available in card form from Garrard Publishing Co., Champaign, Ill. 61820. Copyright 1948.

Page 235: "95 Commonest Nouns" by E. W. Dolch. Available in card form entitled "Picture Word Cards" from Garrard Publishing Co., Champaign, Ill. 61820. Copyright 1941.

Page 236: "1-60 Verbal Opposites" from *Detroit Tests of Learning Aptitude* by H. Baker and B. Lealand (Indianapolis, Ind.: Bobbs-Merrill Co.). Copyright © 1935.

Editor: Antonio Padial
Designer: Paul Quin
Illustrator: Joyce Zavarro
Cover designer: Al Burkhardt

ISBN-0-8224-2500-9 (hardbound)

ISBN-0-8224-2501-7 (paperbound)

Library of Congress Catalog Card Number: 78-75216

Printed in the United States of America.

1.9 8 7 6 5 4 3 2

Contents

Appendixes

Surveys and Forms

Lessons

Figures

Tables

Preface

For many years I have worked with learning-disabled children and young adults in a variety of settings. Much of this work has been done in classrooms, special clinics, and resource centers; in camps and hospitals; and through community organizations and groups.

After some time and much varied experience, my thoughts about learning and behavior disorders have changed. Over the last dozen years or so, I have become an advocate of the developmental point of view. I am increasingly convinced that all persons grow and learn in accord with their own biogenetic timetables.

Yet this natural maturational process may be furthered by education. It may also be frustrated by a lack of appropriate stimulation or training. Learning-disabled persons are those who are not achieving what might reasonably be expected of them once one considers their unique abilities, interests, skills, and constitutional-biological predispositions.

Dyslexia is a learning disability that results in significant reading difficulties. It has been defined as a complex syndrome of associated psychoneurological deficiencies that may include disturbances in orientation, time, written language, spelling, memory, auditory and visual perception, motor skills, and related sensory abilities.

A growing body of research has begun to substantiate that a dyslexic child suffers from maturational delay and unusually slow development of the neuropsychological functions essential for reading. This developmental delay or impairment results in the inability to translate sounds into letter symbols and to comprehend written material. Most authorities agree that the major impairment is not faulty recognition or discrimination but rather the inability to interpret symbols. Many children with severe reading disabilities caused by perceptual-linguistic distortions make reversals or mirror images of letters, words, and symbols — a condition considered a diagnostic sign of dyslexia.

The main purpose of this book is to convey some understanding of current research to teachers, parents, therapists, and other educators of dyslexic children. I believe that if all concerned can understand more fully current theory and research findings, they will be in a better position to help dyslexic persons to learn.

Throughout this book I have emphasized the practical applications of existing knowledge. In the first chapters of Part I, dyslexia is defined in some detail. The neuropsychological brain functions are discussed as they relate to learning and reading processes. The next portion treats the process of language acquisition, and dyslexia is discussed as one form of language disability. A systematic approach to diagnostic methods and techniques is presented next with stress on the functional educational use of test results.

The greater part of this book, Part II, reviews selected neuropsychological approaches to the education of dyslexic children. Certain sensory-motor, visual, auditory, and multisensory learning methods are discussed in detail with illustrative lessons. Chapter 12 gives a short annotated list of instructional materials that may prove especially helpful to those establishing remedial programs. (See the Appendixes for a list of all instructional materials that appear anywhere in the text, even if they are mentioned only in connection with findings reported by a researcher; another list gives names and addresses of suppliers of instructional materials) A special chapter discusses how to increase attention and motivation in dyslexic children; another suggests how to teach dyslexic children to improve their thinking skills. The book also presents a critique of traditional school and clinical organization and offers several alternatives that should enable dyslexic children to learn more effectively. The final chapter considers prognosis and how we might profit from current and emerging research and practice in the education of dyslexic children.

To many readers this may be a controversial book. I have attempted to review and summarize the literature, but this process has been highly selective. Many readers may feel that important studies have been omitted or treated superficially. Since I was trained as an educational psychologist and not as a neurologist or a language or reading specialist, I chose to limit certain chapters. The reader is urged to supplement this book with material from other disciplines.

With increasing public concern about children who are not reading adequately, we can be assured that our schools will be devoting more time and attention to this problem. Dyslexic children will undoubtedly profit from the creation of new preventive plans and from the organization of developmental, remedial, and supplemental prescriptive-teaching programs. As research accumulates we will eventually be able to determine what practices and methods are most effective for educating dyslexic children.

There is good reason to believe that children with severe reading disorders can be educated much more effectively than they have been in the past. What we require is the will and the determination to implement new programs in our schools. My hope is that this book might contribute to the development of better educational programs for dyslexic children. My gratitude is extended to all those persons who are striving to improve the education of dyslexic students and others with specific learning disabilities.

Robert E. Valett, Ed.D.

PART ONE

Neuropsychological
Foundations of Reading

ꓥИꙅdᎮxu Sleꙅdb ᎦꓵH ᓙz sꙅ ꓲDꓘ ɘꓒɿꓑ d

There is an art of reading,
as well as an art of thinking
and an art of writing.
Isaac D'Israeli

CHAPTER ONE

Dyslexia
and Reading Disabilities

Most persons would agree that teachers should be proficient in the arts of reading, thinking, and writing and that their primary function is to develop these skills in their students. Both reading and clear thinking develop with experience, education, and continued practice. Unfortunately many children fail to grasp even the basic skills, and the problem of reading disabilities continues to be of widespread concern.

One report from the U.S. Office of Education indicates that as many as twenty million students may suffer from dyslexia and related disorders (Research Conference Report 1967). Dyslexia is most commonly defined as a severe reading disability due to neuropsychological immaturity or dysfunction. However, persons with significant reading problems are not necessarily dyslexic. Whatever the root of the problem, many children have reading difficulties that warrant special attention and instruction, the earlier the better. Studies show a high incidence of severe reading disabilities in most schools. Two frequently quoted early studies by Durrell (1940) show that of 7,130 children surveyed, between 18 and 20 percent of boys were significantly behind in reading and between 9 and 10 percent of girls were equally deficient. The major deficiencies discovered in these studies were:

- failure to understand word meanings and lack of basic associations

1

- inadequate perception of printed words (too rapid introduction with insufficient experience to assure understanding)
- overemphasis on word analysis
- inability to distinguish phonetic elements
- too many fixations in phrase reading

Other studies substantiate Durrell's findings. Hepworth's (1971) report maintains that 25 percent of school children manifest reading retardation. Such retardation calls for special measures to help children focus attention, provide them with perceptual and auditory training, and reduce their anxiety. More conservative reports, such as those of Bond and Tinker (1973), show that between 8 and 15 percent of those surveyed have reading disabilities and need special instruction. All studies concur that at least twice as many boys as girls have significant reading disabilities. In some populations the disproportion is as high as eight boys to every girl. Evidence exists that some 80 percent of reading-disabled children can be helped if they are identified and provided with special instruction in the first or second grades, whereas fewer than 20 percent profit from such instruction if it is begun after the third grade (Goldberg and Schiffman 1972).

There is no question about the prevalence and seriousness of reading disorders in our schools, and yet most children can be taught to improve their reading with appropriate instruction, special treatment, time, and practice.

In this book, we will consider what might be done to improve the instruction of dyslexic children. Although some of the research and much of the methodology to be discussed may also be of value to those concerned with developmental and remedial reading, the emphasis here is on individual prescriptive teaching of those children with severe reading disorders who might reasonably be classified as dyslexics.

THE READING PROCESS

The test of reading ability is the reader's understanding of written material. One's understanding is best determined by the ability to solve practical problems: comprehending road signs, menus, telephone books, advertisements, maps, and application forms as well as understanding the more abstract content of newspapers, magazines, reference materials, and books.

In order to read a person must acquire a number of basic cognitive and perceptual-linguistic skills:

- the ability to focus attention, to concentrate, and to follow directions
- the ability to understand and interpret spoken language in daily life
- auditory memory and sequencing
- visual memory and sequencing
- word-attack (decoding) skills
- structural-contextual analysis of language
- logical synthesis and interpretation of language
- vocabulary development and expansion
- fluency in scanning and reference skills

These skills are taught in all good developmental reading programs, but their complexity is not always fully understood. Chall summarizes the reading process as "perception (word recognition), comprehension and interpretation, appreciation and application" (Chall 1967, p. 54). Two neuropsychologists describe this process in more detail:

> The reading process starts with the visual perception and analysis of a grapheme, passes on to the recoding of graphemes into the corresponding phonetic structures, and ends with the comprehension of the meaning of what has been written.
>
> It is to be kept in mind that reading in its later developmental stages is transformed into a direct, highly automatized process, in which hardly any use of phonetic analysis and synthesis is made, a process based on the direct recognition of the meaning of written words and sometimes of whole phrases (Christensen and Luria 1975, p. 101).

The perceptual-linguistic elements necessary in learning to read can be comprehended more fully if we consider an example. In Table 1 are several foreign words, which you are asked to translate into English.

Unless the reader knows the languages involved, he or she has no frame of reference for decoding the words or for making the necessary

TABLE 1. Foreign Words

	A	B
1	Molim	Citanje
2	Prosim	Branje
3	Ju Lutem	Lexim
4	пожалуйста	чтение

phonetic associations to the graphemes that are perceived. There are four languages represented: number one is Croatian; number two, Slovenian; number three, Albanian; and number four, Russian. In Column A, the English equivalent for all four words is *please;* in Column B, the English equivalent is *reading.* Most readers will be able to approximate the sounds of the first three pairs of words because they are written in roman letters but will not know their meaning. Since the Russian words are written in a form of the Cyrillic alphabet, only persons familiar with it can begin to decode, associate, and understand the graphemes and their meaning.

Of course, pronunciation of words also varies according to regional-cultural dialect, or what is usually referred to as the "common language." This dialect is internalized and applied in the decoding process with varied accents, intonations, and emphases that result in changes in interpretation and meaning. The spoken English of Wales, New England, and the rural South may all be difficult for the native Hawaiian to understand and interpret. Reading begins with linguistic experiences, which are applied in decoding the component graphemes and corresponding phonemes in written language and then integrated into a culturally meaningful syntax and sentence structure. As readers gain education and experience, the process becomes highly automatic and functional, and there is increasing emphasis on the interpretation of higher-order abstractions and their possible referents and meanings.

Reading, then, is a complex form of symbolic learning in which relatively trivial changes in a word may completely alter pronunciation and meaning. It is a process that involves spoken language, attention, motor ability, various kinds of memory, text organization, and mental imagery; a process "in which the pronounceability of a word influences its perception, as do the meaning and structure of the sentence in which the word appears" (Rosinski 1977, pp. 181–82).

The purpose of reading is to understand the meaningful grapheme units (or morphemes) perceived in words and sentences. Because reading draws on the same linguistic competence as speaking and listening, the reading process involves much more than the identification of words. Word meaning is construed from the syntax of sentences, and "if this syntactic pattern is unfamiliar to the reader, the sentence will not be understood (Dale 1972, p. 189). Recent linguistic research suggests that reading should be taught through the introduction of word groups followed by phoneme-grapheme correspondence and reading aloud.

THE DYSLEXIC SYNDROME

As we have seen, reading is a rather complex perceptual-linguistic process that most persons develop rapidly and shape through education. Eventually the reading process is refined into a series of automatic acts that are quickly integrated psychoneurologically to produce meaningful thoughts and behavior. The reading process itself, though, varies among individuals and is dependent upon such factors as age and maturation, sex, heredity, cultural experience, instruction, practice, and motivation. Valett (1978) discusses many of the cognitive abilities intrinsic to reading. But most cognitive abilities are based on fundamental perceptual-linguistic skills such as auditory-visual integration and sequencing. It is in just such basic skills that dyslexic persons are most deficient.

These deficiencies have been clinically specified for some time. In 1917, the Scottish eye surgeon James Hinshelwood detailed the perceptual distortions in children who could not recognize or comprehend printed words. He concluded that the most probable cause of such severe reading disorders is a congenital defect in the brain, affecting visual memory of words and letters. He believed that the problem might be hereditary (Hinshelwood 1917). The treatment suggested by this early researcher was individual diagnostic-prescriptive teaching, dependent on the degree of visual and auditory memory deficiency.

In 1928, another physician, Samuel Orton, published a clinical report further describing the specific perceptual-linguistic distortions in children with severe reading disabilities. Many of these children made reversals and mirror images of letters and words, and Orton suggested that this phenomenon was due to competing images in both hemispheres of the brain because of failure to establish unilateral cerebral dominance and perceptual consistency (Orton 1928). He labeled this condition *strephosymbolia* (reversed symbols), and it is still accepted as a major diagnostic sign of dyslexia. Later, after an intensive ten-year study of language and reading disorders, Orton further concluded that the one common factor in such disabilities was "a difficulty in repicturing or rebuilding in the order of presentation, *sequences* of letters, of sounds, or of units of movement" (Orton 1937, p. 145). He suggested that remediation should emphasize the teaching of syllables, blends, and words in rhythmic patterns and units.

Gradually, the idea that congenital word blindness and strephosymbolia are caused by psychoneurological disorders became widely accepted by physicians, psychologists, and special educators. But the question of what biological and neurological factors are involved in such severe reading problems has sparked much controversy and stimulated considerable research and discussion. On the basis of neurological studies, Drew (1956) states that congenital word blindness exists and is due to the delayed development of the parietal lobes. This delay disturbs gestalt recognition and the integration of visual patterns and results in difficulties in word recognition and interpretation. In another summary of research, the English neurologist Critchley concludes that "the view currently held by most neurologists is that both ambilaterality and dyslexia are the expressions of a common factor, namely *immaturity of cerebral development*" (emphasis mine) (Critchley 1970, p. 70). This immaturity reportedly results in failure to match written letters and words to corresponding spoken forms and is evidenced by visual rotations and reversals, omissions and substitutions, pronunciation and structural analysis problems, and subsequent difficulties in comprehension.

The behavioral disabilities of dyslexic children have been researched in detail by numerous investigators. A widely acknowledged report by de Hirsch (1968) emphasizes the importance of neuropsychological dysfunctions such as poor memory for details, distorted reproduction of spatial configurations, and related visual-motor problems reflecting personal disorganization and distractibility. De Hirsch concludes that both delayed cerebral dominance and language disorders may reflect maturational delay or dysfunction, and that formal reading instruction should be postponed for such children until success is achieved with perceptual-motor and oral language instruction.

Of major importance to special educators is the research of Myklebust and Johnson at Northwestern University. This team defines dyslexia as a complex syndrome of associated psychoneurological dysfunction, such as disturbances in orientation, time, written language, spelling, memory, auditory and visual perception, motor skills, and related sensory abilities (Myklebust and Johnson 1962). They conclude that for educational purposes it is beneficial to recognize two types of dyslexia: auditory and visual. Auditory dyslexics are characterized by significant difficulties in discriminating letter sounds and blends and in remembering sound patterns, sequences, words, directions, and stories (Johnson and Myklebust 1967). Visual dyslexics have difficulty in following and retaining visual sequences and in the visual analysis and integration of puzzles and similar tasks. They also make frequent letter reversals and inversions and easily confuse similar words and letters (Myklebust, 1968). However, most children who are significantly reading-disabled demonstrate both auditory and visual dyslexia even when the deficiency is primarily one or the other (McGrady 1968).

One of the most extensive studies of dyslexic children was made by the psychologist Kasen (1972). Five hundred dyslexic students at the Ellen K. Raskob Learning Institute in Oakland, California, were statistically evaluated. In this group ages ranged from 6 to 17, and boys outnumbered girls by two and one-half to one. The lowest total score on the Wechsler Intelligence Scale for Children (WISC) was 90, the average Verbal Scale score was 104, and the average Performance Scale score was 105. The lowest WISC subtest scaled scores were Digit Span (9.4) and Arithmetic (9.4), whereas the highest subtest scores were Similarities (11.4) and Picture Completion (10.8). The boys had significantly lower Goodenough Draw-A-Person scores (a mean of 94.3) reflecting their relative visual-motor immaturity. Most important is the picture that emerged from the data of dyslexia as a complex syndrome of associated behavioral dysfunctions:

- 67.2 percent of the group had combined visual and visual-motor problems.

- 66.0 percent were evaluated neurologically and found to have clear signs of minimal neurological dysfunction.

- 65.0 percent had anxiety symptoms.

- 44.2 percent had mixed laterality/crossed dominance.

- 39.7 percent had close relatives with learning disabilities.

- 39.6 percent demonstrated delayed speech at eighteen months of age.

- 39.3 percent evidenced nervous habits such as nail biting, tics, enuresis, and so forth.

- 33.2 percent were developmentally or maturationally delayed.

- 26.8 percent had been labeled hyperactive (impulsive, and so forth).
- 22.4 percent had speech impediments such as poor articulation.
- 18.4 percent were hypoactive with unusually slow responses.
- 10.2 percent had significant auditory discrimination problems.

Kasen's is a landmark study and should be carefully considered by all concerned with statistical research on the dyslexic syndrome.

AN INTRODUCTORY EXAMPLE

At this point it may help to illustrate some of the major specific language disabilities of dyslexic children. Louis is of normal intelligence and eleven years and three months old. In preschool he was slow in talking and demonstrated poor coordination. In kindergarten he proved immature and inattentive and soon fell behind the other children in academic achievement. He has a history of being unable to attack words phonetically. He spells and writes poorly and has reversal and laterality problems.

Although Louis is now in the fifth grade, his current language scores show his abilities to be from two to three years below grade level. His reading vocabulary is at the low second-grade level, and his reading comprehension at the low third-grade level. His spelling ability is at the low second-grade level. Other psychoeducational test results show that his auditory perception remains poor. He continues to confuse simple blends, saying *sl* for *cl* and *dr* for *br*. He also tends to be impulsive and has difficulty in visual sequencing and integration and in organizing what he perceives.

Some examples of Louis's work are presented in Figure 1. The drawing of a man is poorly done for a boy this age, as is his printing of the alphabet. He did not know the dates of his birthday or Christmas, and his spelling difficulties are obvious. On a self-concept test Louis indicated many fears and anxieties about school. He feels he cannot do what is expected of him, and he recognizes that he needs much help with his work. He is lacking in self-confidence and needs intensive remedial education if he is to be prevented from developing even more serious learning and emotional problems. However, it should be noted that Louis's psychological test results indicate a good expressive vocabulary and the potential to learn and achieve with proper help.

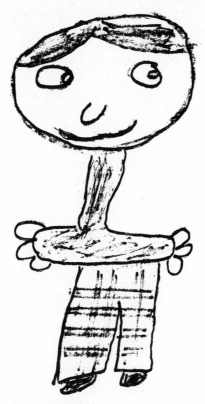

Print your A, B, C's. *ABCDefghigklmnopqrstuvwxyz*

When is your birthday? *Jly 2*

When is Christmas? *acToBer 4*

What I like to do is *pla*

The thing that bothers me is *TesT*

FIGURE 1. An example of work by Louis, a fifth-grade boy

It is tragic that Louis has been passed on from grade to grade without any special help with his language disabilities. Each year he has fallen farther behind; these cumulative deficiencies may have disastrous results. Special auditory, visual, and visual-motor training should have been started when he was in the first grade and continued at his own rate of learning until these basic skills had been mastered. It must be recognized, however, that although Louis demonstrates many of the typical characteristics of the dyslexic child at least he *is* reading at a low level. For every child like Louis, there are many others with similar language problems who never learn to read.

SUMMARY   A large number of persons in our society experience great difficulty in reading and learning. Many of the children in our schools are well below grade level in reading achievement. Some of these children have severe reading disorders that characterize them as dyslexic.

Dyslexia is a disorder that interferes with the meaningful integration of perceptual and linguistic symbols and stems from neuropsychological immaturity or dysfunction. In preschool children of normal intelligence, the disorder usually appears as gross immaturity of psycholinguistic abilities and reading-readiness skills. In school-age children of normal intelligence, a lag of two or more years in reading associated perceptual-linguistic skills usually signals a dyslexic condition.

Dyslexia can be diagnosed and remediated through early intervention and proper treatment. The primary treatment consists of diagnostic-prescriptive teaching that focuses on the neuropsychological processing dysfunction through the use of special instructional methodologies and techniques.

DISCUSSION QUESTIONS AND ACTIVITIES

1. What is the estimated percentage of severe reading disabilities in the public school in your residential area? How does this differ from the percentage for the entire school district?

2. What could be some of the basic causes of the major reading deficiencies described by Durrell?

3. Select another local school and ascertain the ratio of boys to girls with severe reading disabilities.

4. Define *perceptual-linguistic skills*.

5. Discuss what a good reading test might consist of.

6. What is the reason for differentiating between auditory and visual dyslexia?

7. Give an example of strephosymbolia.

8. How does the dyslexic child differ from other children with severe reading disorders?

CHAPTER TWO

Critical Neuropsychological Factors

This chapter presents some of the research findings that support the theory of dyslexia as a neuropsychological processing disorder. Since the major emphasis of this book is on treatment and remediation, the chapter is limited to research that has psychoeducational implications. The studies discussed are comparative and look at the differences, if any, that exist between groups of dyslexic children and groups of non-dyslexic children. Findings will be discussed under the four major topics of general developmental differences, auditory processing differences, visual processing differences, and differences in auditory-visual integration.

GENERAL DEVELOPMENTAL DIFFERENCES

Perhaps the single most striking factor in the history and behavior of eleven-year-old Louis (see Chapter 1) is his general developmental immaturity. His poor reading and language skills are reflections of this lag in growth and maturation. This developmental lag is much more common among boys than girls, as remedial reading specialists and special educators continually reaffirm.

Two developmental studies, conducted by the team of Ilg and

11

Ames, are especially interesting in this regard. They studied hundreds of children between five and ten years of age in Weston and North Haven, Connecticut. Their data support the general supposition that girls of this age group are slightly but consistently ahead of boys in school-readiness skills such as oral language and visual-motor co-ordination; these differences amounted to about six months in favor of girls around the time of school entrance (Ilg and Ames 1965). Ames concludes that the outstanding reason for disturbances in school learning is the immaturity of some children and their unreadiness for the work of the grade in which they have been placed. Research evidence suggests that possibly 50 percent of the children in public school are currently placed one grade above the one in which they can comfortably and effectively do the work. By failing to provide for these tremendous individual and sexual differences in maturity levels, we actually create learning disabilities (Ames 1968).

Gross immaturity in attention, in following directions, and in such basic skills as auditory-visual-motor integration certainly interfere with learning to read. But obviously, there is a tremendous difference between a child who is only six months or so behind and a child who is several years behind in these and other critical skills. The beginning student with significant overt neurological dysfunction is even further handicapped in language and cognitive performance.

One longitudinal study of 390 children between three months and six and a half years old shows that at six and a half, only 76 percent were strongly right-handed, and only 67 percent were homolateral with consistent use of the right hand, foot, and eye (MacBurney and Dunn 1976). However, speech and language test achievement scores significantly favored right-handed children at age nine months, four years, and at six and a half years. Verbal, performance, and full-scale scores on the Wechsler Intelligence Scale for Children (WISC) also favored right-handed children. Furthermore, children whose dominant foot and eye matched their dominant hand (whether right or left) had significantly superior scores. This is representative of the studies suggesting that lateral consistency reflects neuropsychological integration and results in better academic achievement.

Other studies by Dykman, Ackerman, Clements, and Peters (1971) show that learning-disabled children eight and nine years old have significantly greater maturational problems than children ten and eleven. They conclude that neurological immaturity could well explain the attentional problems of such children and that the grade placement system by chronological age used in most schools further compounds their learning problems. Many of these neurological problems appear as lack of control of body parts and functions. Research by Prechtl (1962) shows that of children with choreiform (irregular, spasmodic-involuntary) movements, 90 percent had severe reading problems; among children classified as dyslexics, all had choreiform activity of the eye muscles causing disturbances in fixation and conjugate movements of the eyes. Significantly more (.01 level) children with chorea had learning problems than did those in control groups.

Many other studies show that learning-disabled children with severe reading problems have attentional and control dysfunctions. Some researchers, such as Sheer (1975), refer to these as primary dysfunctions in "focused arousal" with inability to concentrate or attend to relevant associations and with inadequate sequencing of verbal mediation. In these studies, *focused arousal* is defined as selective facilitatory processing; since learning-disabled children show significantly low EEG responses to tone-light stimuli at a frequency length of 40 Hertz, they therefore may not exhibit the cortical excitability necessary for the maintenance of short-term memory. This work indicates that cortical arousal may be enhanced by giving systemic amphetamines, which seem to increase acetylcholine levels in the body and aid in neural transmission. Another relevant summary of research (Rourke 1975) on learning-disabled children suggests that such children, especially when young, have slower visual reaction times. Rourke concludes that cerebral dysfunction is one of the causes of learning disabilities and that cognitive control/field independence dysfunctions are a major problem among seriously retarded readers. In addition to its medical implications, such work has stimulated the use of meditation, yogalike exercises, behavior modification, and biofeedback. Many such psychoeducational activities appear to stimulate EEG activity at 40 Hertz and help develop focused arousal and attentional skills.

A study by Dykstra and Tinney (1969) on sexually correlated differences in specific reading readiness and in first- and second-grade achievement included all boys and girls in eight participating projects of the Cooperative Research Program from schools in four states. Boys made significantly lower scores in visual and auditory discrimination, reading, spelling, and language. Other similar studies abroad (Ekstrand 1976) show that differences by sex in reading and language learning may be due to differences in such brain functions as phonemic recognition; also, nondyslexic males tend to show a right-hemispheric superiority on certain visual discrimination tasks. Developmental differences in young children often go unnoticed until a child has been

exposed to extensive reading instruction in elementary school. Therefore, we will concentrate our discussion on research comparing reading-
disabled/dyslexic children with nondyslexic children when both groups
have been exposed to language and reading programs in school.

BRAIN FUNCTIONS

In order to understand recent research, one must know how the
human brain develops and functions. In the preschool and primary
years, the brain is a plastic organ in which neurological growth,
organization, and integration continue until at least the age of eight.
The brain consists of a left and a right hemisphere; in most individuals
the left hemisphere is dominant. For the purposes of our discussion,
the terms *left* and *right* will be used for *dominant* and *nondominant*.
The reader should be aware, however, that in some individuals (6–8
percent) hemispheric dominance is reversed. Each hemisphere has
major functions that affect the reading process. Figure 2 shows a
schematic drawing of this lateralization of brain function. In most individuals, the right hemisphere is the main center for organizing and
integrating nonverbal, pictorial, and spatial stimuli such as a picture

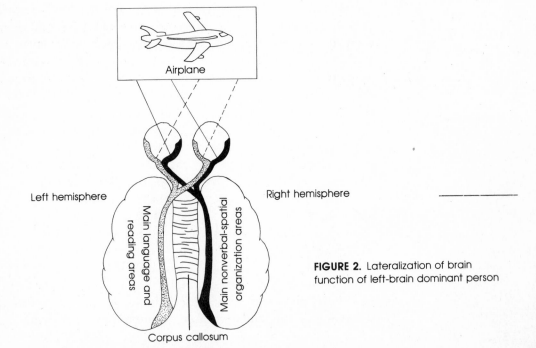

FIGURE 2. Lateralization of brain
function of left-brain dominant person

of an airplane, a face, or an artistic design. The left hemisphere is the primary center for language, words, and symbols. When a child perceives the picture of an airplane on a flash card with the word *airplane,* many processes occur in the child's mind.

First the image on the card is projected on the retina of each eye and passes as an impulse along the optic nerves and across the optic chiasma where most of the nerve fibers cross over to the opposite sides of the brain. The impulse is then transmitted to the visual center located in the occipital lobe at the posterior portion of each cerebral hemisphere. In most persons who are left-brain dominant, visual decoding begins in the right hemisphere with the processing of impulses. The result is the identification and interpretation of a visual gestalt, as, for instance, of an airplane. If the flash card also has the word *airplane* on it, the left hemisphere processes the linguistic symbols presented. Simultaneously, neural impulses are transmitted back and forth across the fibers of the corpus callosum, which connects the two hemispheres. The integration of these varied impulses is a complex neuropsychological act that, if unimpaired, results in the understanding of visual symbols.

Figure 3 is a simplified schematic of the left hemisphere of a left-brain dominant individual. This drawing shows the major brain lobes and association areas of the cerebral cortex of the dominant hemisphere. The frontal lobe contains the areas involved in complex mental acts such as abstract thought and memory as well as motor areas called upon in activities such as writing a letter or playing the piano. The parietal lobe includes areas for tactile-kinesthetic discrimination of such things as geometric forms and common objects. The occipital lobe processes visual stimuli, while the upper part of the temporal lobe

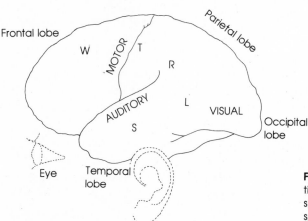

FIGURE 3. Cerebral cortex association areas of dominant left hemisphere, R = reading, L = language, S = speech, W = writing, T = tactual recognition

is concerned with auditory processing and association. Speech is a complex function requiring involvement of the auditory area of the temporal lobe and the speech production area of the frontal lobe. However, reading and other language functions involve both auditory and visual centers in the temporal and occipital lobes.

From this brief introduction to brain functions, we can begin to comprehend the complexity of the reading process. Reading requires numerous perceptual and integrational acts, and it is possible for many dysfunctions to occur in different parts of the brain, in neural structures, or in the biochemical transmission of stimuli between (or within) critical association areas. Such dysfunctions can impair the required integration and organization of whatever is perceived and thereby interfere with the reading process. Differences have been found to exist in critical brain functions between dyslexic and nondyslexic children.

AUDITORY PROCESSING DIFFERENCES

The processing and integration of auditory information is basic to reading. Reading aloud involves both speech and reading areas of the brain. Silent reading demands subvocalization and recall of stored auditory information. One of the first clinical investigators of the interrelationships of these brain functions was the Russian neuropsychologist Aleksandr Luria. On the basis of his work in restoring cognitive functions after brain injury, Luria wrote that although injury to the cortex of the left temporal region does not disturb hearing, the injury nevertheless lessens ability to differentiate sound stimuli. This "disturbance of the phonematic organization of hearing inevitably leads to the disintegration of writing capacity and, within certain limits, to disorders of reading." (Luria 1963, pp. 60-61). In a later investigation of writing and reading disorders, Luria demonstrated that "different types of defects in phonetic analysis and synthesis" occur with a lesion in the posterior division of the left sensory-motor region, and that these are accompanied by a disturbance of the kinesthetic basis of the speech act (Luria 1966, p. 416). Although many other clinical investigators have confirmed that brain lesions can result in auditory and reading disorders, it has been much more difficult to establish that there is dysfunction when lesions are not apparent. Fortunately, however, considerable research has been done in this area.

Zigmond (1966) made a study of sensory processing in nondsylexic and dyslexic children. He found that dyslexic children were inferior in

auditory learning. The auditory functions that most often differen-
tiated the groups were auditory blending and oral spelling. Similar
work on specific auditory perceptual factors by Tallal (1976) shows
that dyslexics suffer from a primary impairment in auditory temporal
processing and that such children are incapable of organizing and integrating stimuli presented at rapid rates, although they can process
the same data at slower rates. This study also suggests that phonic
methods may not be the best initial reading techniques for dyslexic
children.

Recent auditory research with dyslexic children uses dichotic
listening techniques. This process requires simultaneous presentation
of different auditory information to each ear through earphones. For
example, a series of letter sounds and digits such as *1-b-9-m-5* is played
to the right ear while the left ear receives music. The listener is asked to
repeat the letters or digits. The order is reversed to test the other ear.
Although Luria (1963) states that there is no complete representation
of each ear or auditory fibers in the opposite hemisphere (unlike in the
occipital cortex), there is predominant representation in the opposite
hemisphere. Thus, which side of the brain is more proficient may depend on the nature of the auditory input. For numbers, letters, words,
and language sounds, the left hemisphere is usually more proficient.
Therefore, input through the right ear, which transmits this information to the left hemisphere, may be more effective. Surveys such as
those on pages 18 and 19 illustrate another approach to the evaluation
and development of dichotic listening.

In one study by Leong (1976), fifty-eight dyslexic boys with a
mean reading lag of two and a half grades on dichotic digit tasks were
compared with nondyslexic boys. Eight other perceptual processing
tests were also used in this study. Both dyslexics and nondyslexics were
significantly better (.001 level) at processing information through the
right ear than through the left ear. However, dyslexics scored much
lower than nondyslexics, suggesting maturational lag and immaturity
of cerebral development, especially in the synthesis of information.
A series of other studies by Satz (1976) on cerebral dominance and
reading disability shows a correlation between ear and hand dominance and also discloses a right-ear advantage for disabled readers.

Recent research by Van Duyne and Bakker (1976) with primary-
grade children shows developmental changes in auditory processing
and reading patterns. Evidence suggests that early reading is less dependent on dominant-hemisphere (usually left-hemisphere) functioning than advanced reading. In early reading, children tend to show

DICHOTIC LISTENING SURVEY

Student's Name _____ Age _____ Grade _____ Date _____

I. Right Ear Oral Response   Put the earphones on and listen carefully. In your left ear you will hear music. In your right ear you will hear sounds. Repeat the sounds you hear so I can write them down.

2-5_____   b-k_____   fl-st_____   3-1-6_____   m-h-o_____   sp-ed-ic_____

9-4-8-2_____   u-d-a-x_____   en-sh-ly-er_____

Jack had a big dog._____   7-O-5-2-9_____   v-a-l-r-c_____

dr-ing-fl-it-ate_____   The king and queen lived in the palace._____

5-1-6-3-O-2_____   o-g-y-e-n-a_____   fl-er-st-th-ow-dr_____

One of the most interesting birds I ever knew was a bluejay named Jackie. _____

_____   Total REOR errors: _____

II. Right Ear Written Response   Now we will listen to the tape again. But this time I want you to write what you hear in reverse order on this sheet of lined paper. For instance, if you hear 1 - 3 you would write 3 - 1.

2-5_____   b-k_____   3-1-6_____   2-4-9_____   m-h-o_____   s-e-i_____

9-4-8-2_____   u-d-a-x_____   5-3-7-1_____   7-O-5-2-9_____

v-e-l-r-c_____   Total REWR errors:_____

**III. Supplemental
Right Ear Tasks**

Supplemental task errors:_____

Total right ear task errors:_____

continued

IV. Left Ear Oral Response   This time we will change the earphones. You will hear the music in your right ear and the sounds in your left ear. Listen carefully and repeat the sounds you hear so I can write them down.

5-2_____   k-b_____   st-fl_____   1-6-3_____   h-o-m_____   ed-ic-sp_____

4-8-2-9_____   d-a-x-u_____   sh-ly-er-ic_____

Mary had a big doll._____   O-5-2-9-7_____

e-l-r-c-v_____   ing-fl-it-ate-dr_____

The man and woman built a log cabin. _____

1-6-3-O-2-5_____   g-y-e-n-a-o_____   er-st-th-ow-dr-fl_____

A yellow bird with blue wings was on mother's hat._____

Total LEOR errors:_____

V. Left Ear Written Response   This is the last part of the tape. Listen carefully and write down what you hear in reverse order on this other sheet of lined paper.

2-5_____   b-k_____   3-1-6_____   2-4-9_____   m-h-o_____   s-e-i_____

9-4-8-2_____   u-d-a-x_____   5-7-3-1_____   7-O-5-2-9_____

v-e-l-r-c_____   Total LEWR errors:_____

**VI. Supplemental
Left Ear Tasks**

Supplemental task errors:_____

Total left ear task errors:_____

Right Ear Advantage = Total left ear errors minus total right ear errors: _____

Comments:

nondominant-hemispheric (usually right-hemispheric) representation of language through more attention to the visual perceptual figures of the material, and they tend to read more slowly with fewer errors. Later, fluent readers decode much faster using left-hemispheric representation of language, but they tend to make more errors. In other research, Bakker (1968) found left-ear advantage in the recall of nonverbal temporal patterns such as tapped rhythms and sounds. Bakker has also demonstrated that meaningful words, nonsense words, consonants, and vowels can be used as verbal stimuli in dichotic listening tasks. Also of considerable importance for education is the finding that, for most children, syllables spoken in the right ear are better identified than syllables spoken in the left ear.

VISUAL PROCESSING DIFFERENCES

Reading demands focusing of the eyes and coordinated movements of the eye muscles as the eyes scan the page. Muscular incoordination of the eyes may interfere with visual perception. For example, in amblyopia the brain tends to ignore the input of one eye, which has become "lazy" due to muscle weakness (strabismus). Double vision may result from this condition; it is treated by patching the stronger eye (and through the use of glasses, if needed) and developing the weaker eye through sensory training. In addition to ocular pursuit and coordination, visual perception is also influenced by varied sensory stimuli such as print size, color, and the organization of the material on the page.

Our previous consideration of the functional areas of the cerebral cortex (see Figure 3) emphasized that reading involves the decoding and reorganization of auditory, visual, and linguistic symbols. The occipital area of the brain contains a storage area for forms that is linked to other areas, such as the posterior parietal lobe, where patterns such as letters and words are stored; other neural association fibers then connect these areas with the auditory centers and the higher cognitive thought units in the frontal lobes.

Yet another part of the cortex in the occipital area blends the separate images from each eye for binocular vision and depth perception. Reading readiness requires the organization of different sensory systems including the integration of visual data and information experienced through ocular convergence, spatial direction and orientation, and perceptual cues of shadow, color, form, hue, and contextual relationships.

Arthur Linksz, a professor of clinical opththalmology, gives a detailed explanation of the function of the optic nerves and tracts in visual perception and language. Linksz describes the interrelatedness of central brain processes and the primary importance of speech and auditory decoding in reading and writing. He explains the gradual development of phonic decoding and reading as a unique left-brain operation resulting from human evolution. Visual perception is also a developmental skill in which dominance of one eye is acquired through use. Linksz argues that handedness is a prime determinant of eyedness and that "every reasonable effort is justified in trying to redirect left-handed children to write with the right hand" (Linksz 1973, p. 180).

Visual perception and integration is a developmental process that can be modified by experience and training. The gradual effects of such experience can be seen in the slow but continued change in such visual skills as fixation, recognition span, and comprehension. In Table 2 (adapted from Taylor 1966), we see that the average first-grade reader has 240 eye fixations per 100 words, but that fixations are gradually reduced to 83 in high school. Similarly, the first-grade child has an average span of recognition of about half a word, which slowly increases to 1.21 words in high school. As fixations are reduced and recognition span increases, comprehension develops from 75 words a minute in first grade to 298 words a minute in high school.

Findings such as these have had a direct influence on visual training and remedial reading practices. As eye fixation and word recognition span are essentially ocular coordination and organization problems, direct attempts should be made to remediate them. This is commonly done through the use of flash cards and tachistoscopes, or

TABLE 2. Developmental Visual Skills in Reading

	Grade						Junior high	High school	College
	1	2	3	4	5	6			
Average span of recognition in words	.42	.50	.59	.73	.85	.95	1.05	1.21	1.33
Average rate of comprehension per minute	75	100	138	180	216	235	255	298	340
Average fixations per 100 words	240	200	170	136	118	105	95	83	75

Source: E. Taylor, The Fundamental Reading Skill (Springfield, Ill.: Charles C. Thomas), p. 154.

controlled readers. Such training increases the span of recognition, improves accuracy of visual perception, and, as Lawson (1968) points out, helps increase alertness and attention and develop the reader's ability to organize material.

Years ago, Goldstein (1948) showed that many reading disturbances are related to the analysis and synthesis of visual stimuli and that damage to the occipital lobe or related parts of the brain can cause varied and complex visual disorders that interfere with reading. Since then, many other researchers have confirmed this and similar studies on the importance of the visual cortex.

In his work on the development of higher cortical functions in humans, Luria explains that when the visual cortex is damaged, it may be able to deal with only one point of excitation at a time: "In cases of literal (printed letters) alexia, the integrated perception of graphemes and the visual differentiation of those signs with cue value is so disrupted that either the letters lose their meanings altogether or their identification becomes highly unstable" (Luria 1966, p. 426). By increasing the stimulus cue value of certain letters and words (with tactile-kinesthetic material, color, and so forth), perceptual integration can be enhanced. Luria also discovered that the secondary zones of the visual cortex were complex structures that synthesize, code, and organize visual stimuli. Defects in these zones result in the inability to combine individual perceptual units into complete forms. If the defect extends to the reading area of the left hemisphere, confusion of letters with similar configurations results in inversions, reversals, omissions, and distortions. Interestingly, Russian clinicians also discovered that some rapid eye movements and irregular visual perceptions could be overcome in part through the use of caffeine. Their test

Before injection of caffeine

Thirty minutes after injection of caffeine

FIGURE 4. Experiment with caffeine. Note disappearance of the signs of optic ataxia in a patient with a bilateral wound of the anterior zones of the occipital region after injection of caffeine. Tests require placing a dot in the center of a circle and a cross, and tracing outlines. Source: Figure 32 from The Working Brain: An introduction to Neuropsychology, by A. R. Luria, © Penguin Books Ltd. 1973, translation © Penguin Books Ltd. 1973, Basic Books, Inc., Publishers, New York.

subjects showed substantial improvement in visual perceptual attention and coordination within a thirty-to-forty minute period after caffeine was given. One dramatic example of the biochemical influences
on visual-motor behavior is presented in Figure 4.

Many similar kinds of visual coordination, analysis, and integration problems are found in children without obvious lesions or history
of traumatic injury to the occipital areas. This leads to the supposition
that a minimal form of cerebral dysfunction exists that also disrupts
neural transmission and integration of perceptual units. This disrup-
tion may be caused by poor or immature neural development or
biochemical inadequacies. One early summary of neurological factors
in familial congenital word blindness (Drew 1956) concludes that an
inherited factor caused delayed development of the parietal lobes and
thus disturbed gestalt recognition of visual patterns and resulted in
word blindness and associated reading disabilities. Obviously, schools
and clinics must consider the possibility of such biological factors when
they place children in reading programs.

Recent investigations by Frank and Levinson (1975–1976) have
resulted in their radical redefinition of dyslexia as a cerebellar-
vestibular dysfunction, with resulting subclinical nystagmus and control problems in ocular fixation and sequential screening. In one study
of more than 1,000 children, they determined the etiology to be a
genetic-biochemical dysfunction of the labyrinthine vestibular-
cerebellar circuitry, ear infections, and a stimulus deprivation or inadequate perceptual-motor input. In other studies (Frank and Levinson 1976) these workers found that of 72 dysmetric dyslexic children
referred for blind electronystagmography (measurement of the rapid
involuntary oscillations of the eyeballs), 85 percent evidenced some
vestibular abnormality. In another study of 250 dyslexic children, 97
percent were found to have cerebellar-vestibular dysfunctions that
decreased their visual tracking capacity. These researchers feel that
cerebellar-vestibular problems are the primary cause of dyslexia.
Although these studies are controversial, other evidence (see Chapter
3) indicates that the cerebellum plays a vital role in the organization
and orientation of sensory stimuli that contribute to visual decoding
and reading. Impaired orienting and visual tracking may be due, in
part, to inadequate cerebellar and vestibular functioning. Ocular fixation and scanning exercises, together with rhythmic cerebellar-
vestibular development activities and medication may be indicated
and are discussed below.

Much psychoeducational research has been done on the importance of visual tracking and perceptual span in reading. Some of

Taylor's work in this area was presented earlier in this chapter. Long ago, in a series of experiments, Gray (1922) found that older and better readers have fewer eye movements per line, shorter pauses, and fewer regressive movements. He found that reading rate and comprehension are both positively correlated to the length of the span of perception. Related tests by Goins (1958) disclosed that visual closure and perceptual speed or the ability to perceive visual stimuli rapidly are the most significant factors in reading ability.

Considerable work has been done with dyslexic children using such instruments as the Illinois Test of Psycholinguistic Abilities (ITPA). In one such study on the psychological correlates of severe reading disability, Kass (1962) found that dyslexic children had greater difficulty than nondyslexic controls in reproducing visual symbols, predicting a whole from parts, duplicating a visual image from memory, and comparing detailed figures rapidly. Another similar neuropsychological investigation of thirty-nine boys with developmental dyslexia disclosed that reading dysfunction is highly correlated to poor performance on visual and verbal tasks requiring the sequential processing of material (Doehring 1968).

Dyslexic children, then, do have significantly greater visual tracking, integration, and processing problems than nondyslexic children. But these difficulties are seldom seen without related auditory and visual-motor problems. Accordingly, most research has focused on determining differences in what is usually referred to as "auditory-visual integration."

DIFFERENCES IN AUDITORY-VISUAL INTEGRATION

Jastak and Jastak (1976, p. 90) state that reading is a process of transcoding a series of visual-kinesthetic symbols into vocal or subvocal sound sequences and that in the dyslexic the connections between visual centers and related language areas of the left hemisphere are interrupted as a result of vascular defects. Because complex behavioral processes such as reading are in fact not localized, but distributed in broad areas of the brain, the contribution of each cortical zone to the organization of the whole is relatively specific (Christensen 1975). Because dyslexia is essentially a handicap of sensory integration due to neuropsychological dysfunction and leading to communication problems, learning is aided through systems of multisensory feedback and compensation.

The work of Satz and Van Nostrand (1973) presents psychometric evidence of a left-hemispheric lag in the auditory-visual integrative skills of dyslexic children. These findings have been substantiated in repeated studies over many years. In one notable experiment, Katz and Deutsch (1963) gave first-, third-, and fifth-grade children a number of visual, auditory, memory, and reaction-time tests. Test results demonstrated that poor readers showed much greater difficulty in discriminating between qualitatively different visual and auditory stimuli, while older poor readers, faced with more complex reading tests, performed worst on tasks integrating auditory-visual stimuli. Similar results were obtained by Birch and Belmont (1964) in a comparison of auditory-visual integration skills in two hundred readers. Reading-disabled children had significantly lower auditory-visual performance, and the researchers conclude that these skills are essential factors in the reading process.

An interesting study of the specific reading disabilities of 203 fifth-grade children is reported by Mariam (1966). All of these children were given the Lorge-Thorndike Intelligence Tests (and found to be of normal mental ability), Iowa Tests of Basic Skills, and the Silent Reading Diagnostic Tests. In addition they were tested for neurological organization, which included laterality of eye-hand-foot, creeping patterns, touching thumb to forefinger, and supination and pronation of the palms. Sixty-nine percent of these children had problems in visual-auditory recognition, reading comprehension, and oral reading. Interestingly, there was also a high proportion of mixed laterality, but no significant differences in the ability to attack words phonetically.

Similarly, Owen, Adams, Forrest, Stolz, and Fisher (1971) administered special neurological examinations to seventy-six children of normal intelligence but with significant reading disability. They found convincing evidence of immaturity in the ordering and sequencing of auditory stimuli such as sound patterns tapped in rhythm. Another study by Corkin (1974) on the serial-ordering problems of seriously retarded readers suggests that although efficiency in remembering serial position of integrated auditory-visual stimuli increased with age, average readers surpassed inferior readers at all ages studied. Other significant differences on WISC Arithmetic and Digit Span subtests between learning-disabled and nondisabled children have been found by Ackerman, Peters, and Dykman (1971) and interpreted as evidence of a basic inability of the learning-disabled to hold sensory data until they can be processed, integrated, and synthesized.

A recent major report by Witelson (1976) shows that developmentally dyslexic boys may have an abnormal right-hemisphere specialization for spatial processing and integration. In this study, 85 dyslexic boys were compared with 156 controls. All subjects were between six and fourteen years of age. The dyslexic youngsters showed statistically significant deficiencies in the following skills: right-hemispheric visual processing of tachistoscopic figures, left-hemispheric auditory processing of dichotic listening tasks, and tactile identification of shapes. Witelson concludes that these dyslexic boys lacked normal neural organization in both spatial processing and in auditory-linguistic functioning and integration. Such evidence of developmental delays in brain functioning and organization indicates that priority might best be given to visual-spatial processing training in young children. Auditory-linguistic training perhaps should be delayed until such children reach a more advanced stage of neuropsychological maturity.

Related psychophysiological studies by Hughes (1976) indicate that dyslexia may be a systemic disorder. He found abnormal monoanime oxidase and thyroxine levels in his subjects. The findings suggest biochemical electrolyte imbalance with resulting central nervous system neurotransmission dysfunction. Similar implications are to be found in the abnormal metabolic and other physiological responses discovered by Levine (1976) in poor readers with auditory-visual integration problems.

SUMMARY

Considerable clinical and experimental evidence indicates that dyslexic children do, in fact, have some significant auditory, visual, and integrational processing deficiencies. Such neuropsychological deficiencies must be considered in any educational or remedial plan for dyslexic children. However, the need for continued research is great. Undoubtedly, future studies will produce fuller understanding of brain function and the reading process, but an objective consideration of available research must lead to the conclusion that *developmental* dyslexia is a reality.

Although it may be a long time before existing studies can be fully confirmed and their results clearly understood, they do present immediate possibilities for further research and psychoeducational practice. The obvious practical indications are for developmental diagnosis, placement, and the neuropsychological education and treatment of dyslexic children. The immediate educational need is for innovative teaching that will improve their auditory, visual, and neuropsychological integration and performance.

DISCUSSION QUESTIONS AND ACTIVITIES

1. In what ways are girls readier to read than boys?

2. Outline two ways that schools might be organized to accommodate developmentally immature children.

3. How do the right and left hemispheres of the brain vary in reading functions?

4. What is the function of the dominant temporal region of the brain?

5. Summarize some of the research findings that differentiate dyslexic from nondyslexic children.

6. Select and discuss a research article on visual training for severe reading disorders.

7. Create a set of lowercase letters with high-stimulus cue value.

8. How might biochemical influences positively affect the reading process?

9. What is a cerebellar-vestibular dysfunction and how might it influence behavior?

10. Give some examples of intersensory integrative functions.

11. How do Witelson's findings about differences in dyslexic boys differ from most other findings?

The surprising prevalence
of reading disabilities
and their frequent association
with minimal birth injuries
tend to support our thesis
that these injuries
are more common
than is ordinarily supposed.

Arnold Gesell

CHAPTER THREE

Neuropsychological Functions

Cerebral dysfunction is often apparent in dyslexics and interferes with the processing of sensory information. The dysfunction can occur in one or several areas of the brain. It is helpful for the special educator to have some knowledge of these brain units and systems.

BASIC NEUROPSYCHOLOGY

Luria (1973) describes three major functional units of the brain that are involved in any higher form of mental activity. One unit is concerned with regulating, activating, and modulating neural impulses. A second unit obtains, processes, and stores information from the outside world. The third unit is mainly concerned with the programming and verification of cognitive operations. Each functioning unit comprises several organs or cortical areas that together constitute a neuropsychological system.

Higher mental processes are not static or completely localized and are especially fluid during the early years of development. The processes required in reading include distinguishing the essential features of a linguistic symbol (decoding), searching for corresponding information (analysis), comparing the features with each other (synthesis), creating an appropriate hypothesis as to the meaning (conjecture), and evaluating these elements (verification). Since a disturbance in brain function in infancy or early childhood inevitably results in the incomplete development of the higher cognitive areas, the reading process may be seriously impaired. Each of the three functional units is outlined in Table 3 and will be considered separately.

Regulation. One regulating unit, called the reticular activating system, is concerned with such essential psychophysiological elements as arousal, attention, control, memory, and time orientation. The grossly immature child who cannot focus his or her attention and energies on a task may require special developmental training in these areas before he or she begins to read.

The reticular activating system consists of neural fibers extending along the spinal cord and medulla oblongata to the midbrain and the cerebral cortex. This nerve net controls and modulates neural tone and excitation and is responsible for focused arousal.

Another kind of brain regulation takes place through the vestibular and proprioceptive systems, which are responsible for orientation and integration of incoming data from exterior sources. The

TABLE 3. Neuropsychological Functions

Interrelated brain units	Systems	Anatomic structure	Activating sources
Regulation:			
Arousal and attention	Reticular activating	Spinal cord	Metabolic
Facilitation and inhibition		Medulla oblongata	
Memory and time orientation	Vestibular and proprioceptive systems	Cerebral cortex Cerebellum	General stimulation
Processing:			
Sensory reception and analysis			
Spatial organization	Cortical association areas	Left and right cerebral hemispheres:	Specific sensory input and manipulation
Schematic symbolization		visual (occipital)	
Coding and memory		auditory (temporal)	
Sensory-perceptual integration		sensory (parietal)	
Programming:			
Goal orientation and planning	Great pyramidal tract	Motor cortex	Thinking: conscious intent
Synthesis and execution			
Verification	Prefrontal cortical areas	Frontal lobes	internal speech
Correction			feedback

sensory receptors in the ear and the skin are the major external parts of this system, which centers in the brainstem but includes such organs as the thalamus and the cerebellum. Research reported by Fishbein (1976) indicates that two brain structures greatly modified by human evolution are the thalamus and hippocampus, which are essentially responsible for emotional states and control. Neural fibers running from the prefrontal lobes of the cortex to the thalamus and brain stem also form part of the total system through which higher cognitive plans and intentions affect the reticular formation.

Only recently has the importance of the cerebellum in the learning process been understood. The cerebellum is one of the parts of the central nervous system concerned with coordinated movement. John Eccles, the Nobel-prize-winning neurophysiologist, states that we should think of the cerebellum as the organ that "is designed to function as a computer in handling all the complex inputs from receptors or from other parts of the brain" (Eccles 1972, p. 120). Although the cerebral cortex is the command center of the brain, the cerebellum contains the computational machinery necessary to regulate movement and to produce complex actions. Eccles has also described how this computational output is entirely regulated by the inhibitory function of special cells affected by learning: ". . . in the process of learning, neuronal activation leads first to specific RNA synthesis and this, in turn, to protein synthesis and so finally to synaptic growth and the coding of memory" (Eccles 1972, p. 183).

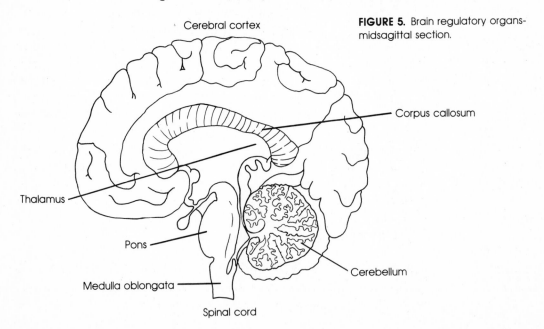

FIGURE 5. Brain regulatory organs-midsagittal section.

Cerebral cortex

Corpus callosum

Thalamus

Pons

Cerebellum

Medulla oblongata

Spinal cord

Although brain function develops in accord with genetic instructions, it is important to note that the speech and reading areas are created in *readiness* for learning a language. All cultural and linguistic material is learned and has demonstrable structural and functional effects on the brain as evidenced by actual microstructural changes in brain tissue as learning takes place. A number of neurophysiological changes due to learning are documented in this chapter and summarized later on. Sensory-motor adaptation is the most basic form of learning that affects the regulatory unit of the brain. Since the primary cerebellar function is that of integrating and regulating motor output, some researchers hypothesize that "certain kinds of vestibular *stimulation* especially, and possibly some of the afferent flow up from the spinal column may result in lowering the excitatory state of the reticular formation through cerebellar inhibition" (Ayres 1972b, p. 49). Research by Ayres and others indicates that sensory-motor learning may improve cerebellar inhibition and reduce incoordinate movements such as poor visual focusing and tracking.

These and other findings reported in this chapter have stimulated investigation into therapeutic intervention and treatment of regulatory-unit dysfunctions. Since biochemical and metabolic actions appear to be the primary stimulators in basic neuropsychological systems and units, a great deal of current research focuses on nutritional and biochemical intervention. Of more interest to special educators and psychologists, however, are the findings that sensory-motor stimulation and learning may help to overcome some higher-order academic problems such as reading disability. It appears that sensory-motor stimulation may change the afferent neurophysiological field in such a way that the immature or damaged system is bolstered and restored through the additional proprioceptive impulses leading to improved biochemical interaction, neural growth, and improved performance. The schematic drawing of brain regulatory organs (Figure 5) illustrates areas involved in the regulatory unit—all of which are affected by biochemical interaction and learning. The pons and the medulla oblongata, located in the hindmost part of the brain, are concerned with such regulatory functions as breathing, heartbeat, and blood pressure; the other regulatory areas have already been discussed. The effects of learning and specific remedial education are even more profound on the processing and programming units of the brain.

Processing.   The processing unit of the brain consists of specific cortical regions in the left and right hemispheres as well as the corpus callosum that connects the hemispheres. If we look again at Figure 3, illustrating the cerebral cortex association areas, we can see that the posterior associative center of the cortex is primarily involved in processing symbolic information.

Actual sensory reception and analysis of data goes on in both hemispheres, but with different priorities and goals. Spatial organization, such as integrating block designs, gesturing, and drawing three-dimensional designs, have been shown by researchers such as Bogen, Fisher, Vogel (1965) and Galin and Ornstein (1972) to be largely right-hemispheric functions. On the other hand, symbolization and the learning of language are largely left-brain processes. However, studies show that in the brain functions of severe epileptics who have undergone surgical disconnection of the hemispheres by severing the corpus callosum, even the disconnected minor hemisphere "is able to comprehend both written and spoken words to some extent, although this comprehension cannot be expressed verbally" (Sperry 1968, p. 731). Research indicates that both hemispheres tend to develop equally at about the same rate without significant differentiation of functions until the age of five or six. Specialization occurs after this age.

Processing of stimuli requires the coding, storage, and integration of sensory-perceptual information, but the integration of data requires the transmission and interchange of coded neural impulses between the left and right hemispheres through the corpus callosum. Gazzangia (1967, p. 29) explains that

> visual pattern information can be transmitted through the corpus callosum . . . a copy of the visual world as seen in one hemisphere is sent over to the other . . . somewhere and somehow all or part of the callosum transmits not only a visual scene but also a complicated neural code of a higher order.

Although the work of Sperry conclusively demonstrates that division of the corpus callosum resulted in memory defects and serious integrational dysfunctions, it also shows that the minor hemisphere does have some language potential that can be developed with specific training. Less radical damage to the corpus callosum can result in processing disorders and confusion. Moreover, lesion of the fibers of the anterior zones of the corpus callosum disconnects symmetrical points of the premotor and motor cortex and impairs the smooth and coordinated movements of both hands, resulting in drastic effects on behavior (Luria 1973, p. 254). Experimental work by Levy (1967, 1972) demonstrates that a person may have difficulty in dealing with data from one hemisphere because of interference from the other, thus further emphasizing the importance of neural transmission and integration.

Some of this work may have educational implications. Ayres (1972a) argues that, since disorders in the integration of auditory, vestibular, and somatosensory stimuli may interfere with language development, improving communication between the two brain hemispheres by transcallosal development and strengthening should be especially important for reading. Special learning activities such as spatial-symbolic games and other sensory-integrative tasks may strengthen communication between cortical hemispheres. Similar suggestions have been made by Whittrock (1975), who proposes new strategies for teaching children to associate sounds and semantic meanings of words (usually in the left hemisphere) with the recognition and integration of their shapes (usually in the right hemisphere).

Programming. We now come to a consideration of the third major brain unit involved in reading and higher-order cognitive functioning. This unit is responsible for programming data. Programming, of course, depends on the prior reception, regulation, and processing of incoming sensory data and remains closely dependent on and interrelated with these other functions.

The cognitive operations involved are planning and executing personal goals. Luria (1973) stresses the importance of plans and intentions on neuropsychological functioning. As an example, the intention to read is seldom a response to an external stimulus, such as a book. Instead, the intention to read creates a model scheme of future needs and of what the human organism must do to achieve them. Psychoneurological impulses, and the acts and movements stemming from them, are shaped, in part, through complex conscious actions dictated by goals and intentions formed through speech and thought.

The organs involved in programming are the frontal lobes and the motor cortex of the brain. The frontal lobes are concerned with ideation, conscious intent, and internalized speech. Much of spoken language is controlled by the motor cortex and modified through feedback providing verification and correction of linguistic expression. The great pyramidal tract is a system of cells whose impulses are carried from the motor cortex through the spinal cord to the muscles. These motor impulses are controlled through interacting neural systems of dendrites and glia. The prefrontal area of the brain has connections with all other systems and exerts executive control.

Much of the recent work in cognition is being used in neuropsychological education. For instance, Meichenbaum (1976) describes cognitive-conceptual performance tasks and linguistic learning strategies that should be used with learning-disabled children. Other researchers describe a variety of cognitive development programs for children who have not been taught to think. For example, Levin and Allen (1976) report on cognitive development strategies and programs to teach children to read. All of these psychoeducational strategies emphasize subvocal speech (or talking to oneself) as an important activator of such programming operations as synthesizing information and planning a course of action.

NEUROPHYSIOLOGICAL CHANGES

Neurological growth and development cause a number of changes in the brain and nervous system. Education is a form of guided experience that results in behavior changes. Sensory and perceptual education produces neuropsychological changes that may aid the cognitive integration required in such mental operations as reading.

Neural stimuli are transmitted in the form of electrochemical impulses from the axon of one neuron to the dendrite of the next. In passing from one neuron to another, the impulse crosses a synapse, the area that lies between two neurons. Neurons vary in shape and structure according to their location in the body. Figure 6 is a schematic drawing

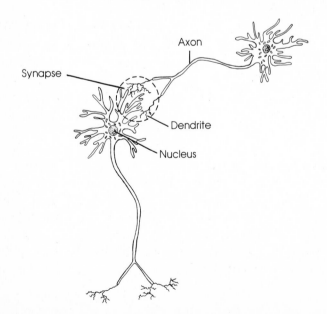

FIGURE 6. Neuron from the cerebral cortex

of a neuron from the cerebral cortex. Impulses proceed along the axon to a dendrite, which passes them across the synapse. The synapse undergoes a biochemical change as the impulse is passed and offers resistance. However, with repetition and training, habit patterns develop that lower the resistance at the synapses (Greisheimer 1945). In this way new connections are formed that promote the elongation and growth of neural fibers and the biochemical modification of synaptic areas.

Donald Hebb, an early neuropsychologist, believed metabolic change triggered by repeated firing of neural cells develops synaptic knobs that enhance neurological integration: "When an axon of cell A is near enough to excite a cell B and repeatedly or persistently takes part in firing it, some growth process or metabolic change takes place in one or both cells such that A's efficiency, as one of the cells firing B, is increased" (Hebb 1949, p. 62). Hebb further suggested that these changing cells are gradually assembled into complex sequences that are the root structure of cognition. Later, Hebb, Lambert, and Tucker (1973) explained how perceptual and sensory learning tasks may initiate complex central activity in the nervous system and produce changes in cortical transmission paths that lead to the appearance and refinement of human language.

The extensive work of other researchers substantiates that neuronal connections develop as a result of learning. Eccles, Ito, and Szentagothai (1967, p. 314) suggest that "in the learning of movements and skills there is the microgrowth of neural organization giving increased synaptic function."

Other studies, such as those by Ingvar and Schwartz (1974), show that speech and reading activate the blood-flow pattern in the premotor, the middle and lower rolandic, and the anterior and middle sylvian region of the dominant hemisphere. Therefore both neurophysiologic and physiologic changes enable the brain to adapt and provide corrective responses that result in appropriate problem-solving behavior.

Several studies demonstrate that highly specific changes in the brain occur as a result of perceptual-motor learning and environmental influences. In one such study (Krech, Rosenzweig, and Bennett 1962) young rats were given thirty days of free maze play including "toys" and sensory-motor stimulation. The rats significantly increased their discriminatory and problem-solving abilities, and on dissection showed changes in brain morphology and biochemistry. In a later study (1966) the same investigators reported that rats held in enriched environments have heavier brains and healthier bodies than rats held in restricted environments.

Perhaps the most important study of this kind was reported by the team of Diamond, Law, Rhodes, Lindner, Rosenzweig, Krech, and Bennett (1966) at the University of California, Berkeley. Twenty-one pairs of littermate rats were divided into an experimental "environmental complexity and training group" and a separate control group; after eighty days of training, their brains were removed and slides were made that showed experimental training had resulted in a 6.4 percent increase in the depth of the visual cortex and a 14 percent greater glia to neuron ratio.

Altman and Dos (1966), studying the effects of motor exercise on the brain chemistry of rats, found an increase in the incorporation of radioactive leucine into the neuronal protein. This finding was reconfirmed by Hydén and Lange (1970) when they showed that rats increased in both leucine and hippocampal neurons after handedness-transfer training. More recently, other researchers have found photomicroscopic evidence of axon sprouting from intact nerve cells near damaged parts of rat brains. These findings suggest that glial cell growth is influenced by biochemical regulators of large molecular weight, which make the cells grow "in a quite dramatic fashion" (Pines 1977). One explanation of these findings is that synaptic transmission and neural growth occurs through chemical mediation by a substance called acetylcholine (Ach), which is released from nerve terminals by calcium. Synaptic transmission is also very sensitive to toxic substances assimilated by the brain (Eccles 1972).

SUMMARY

The regulation and control of neural impulses is largely a brain operation involving the reticular and vestibular systems. The cerebellum serves as an integration and relay center in this operation. Decoding and processing of information occur in the appropriate areas of the cerebral cortex. In most persons, the left-hemispheric association areas are the processing centers for language, but data are transmitted between the two sides of the brain through the corpus callosum. Programming is a conscious act effected through the frontal lobes and the motor cortex area of the brain.

Reading requires the regulation, processing, and programming of neural impulses, perceptions, and cognitions. Changes occur in the brain during the process of learning to read. Of major importance is the neural growth that occurs at synaptic junctions where chemical neurotransmitters are affected by training and practice.

Considerable evidence exists that brain growth and functioning are significantly affected by both biochemistry and education. Biochemical alterations in neuropsychological functions can be effected through nutrition and the administration of mind-altering drugs. Sensory, perceptual, and psycholinguistic training also causes neural growth and change. Neuropsychological education improves the regulation, processing, and programming units of the brain and furthers total neurological growth and cognitive operations such as reading.

DISCUSSION QUESTIONS AND ACTIVITIES

1. Describe the active perceptual processes required in reading.

2. Discuss the function and relationship of the vestibular system to reading.

3. What is the reticular activating system and how does it function?

4. Which brain center is primarily involved in processing symbolic data comprising "reading"?

5. Differentiate between left- and right-brain functions and their contributions to the reading process.

6. How might a defective corpus callosum interfere with reading?

7. Create a spatial-symbolic game and demonstrate its possible use in strengthening hemispheric and sensory integration.

8. Describe what organs are involved in the programming unit and their importance for reading.

9. Discuss the process of synaptic neurotransmission and how it might be brought about by special education.

10. Discuss Hebb's cell assembly theory.

11. Evaluate a current research article on the effects of learning on neural growth and development.

CHAPTER FOUR

Language Acquisition

Human language is a complex system of communication, continuously evolving as each human being interacts with others and with the environment, drawn on by the *desire* to express thoughts and feelings. A child begins very early to associate sounds with meaning. Gradually, the sounds the child makes are refined into words and combined into sentences. While still quite young, the child is expected to learn written symbols representing these sounds. If these associations are learned well enough, reading takes place. It is important to understand that reading is an advanced linguistic process of decoding and attributing meaning.

Within this context, dyslexia can be defined as a specific language disability. The foundations of reading are the basic sensory and perceptual-linguistic skills. Since the remediation of severe reading disorders invariably begins with a return to more fundamental language skills, these skills and abilities will be discussed in some detail here.

SPECIFIC LANGUAGE ABILITIES

Three major linguistic abilities are essential to communication: the receptive ability; the mediational-associative-integrational ability; and the expressive ability. Each of these needs to be understood and considered in any developmental or remedial language program. The psychoneurological processes involved are described by Myklebust (1965) and others, and will be summarized here.

Receptive Language Ability.   The auditory, visual, and kinesthetic-motor channels to the central nervous system must be intact and functional for a child to hear, see, feel, and get in touch with the environment. It is obvious that a child who is hard of hearing or whose vision is impaired will have problems in "tuning in" on the environment and may therefore be slow in acquiring essential information.

But when a child has less obvious sensory and perceptual problems she or he may be misunderstood rather than helped to overcome them. Many children arrive at school still too immature to focus their attention. Many psychologists, such as Jensen (1969), have demonstrated that without an attention span long enough to listen to and understand information and directions, a child cannot learn.

With many dyslexic children, one must begin by improving such receptive language skills as relating, focusing, listening, and receiving. Most researchers and clinicians would agree with Bannatyne (1968) that speech and language training of dyslexic children should begin with "emotive communication" involving art, music, and movement along with conversation. Later, training in the discrimination and processing of phonetic sounds and sequences can be introduced. Formal reading follows.

Mediational-Associative-Integrational Ability.   Mediational abilities are those neuropsychological processes that occur between the reception of information and its eventual expression in overt behavior. The critical mediational abilities are those of memory storage, comprehension, association and coding, symbolic sorting and discrimination, analysis, and synthesis. These are often referred to as "thinking skills."

Mediational language involves carrying on an internal conversation with oneself, thereby creating relationships between external sounds and objects, and the symbolic representations of the mind. Mediational language is a covert mental activity that is acquired by learning such skills as subvocalization of attributes, names, or classifications.

Some researchers have suggested ways to develop mediational language in children. Kaplan-Fitzgerald (1977) describes how severely language-handicapped children can often think and express themselves more fully when they use sign language along with speech in labeling and naming things. Caldwell and Hall (1969) demonstrate that concept training relates to letter discrimination: in their study with seventy-two kindergarten children, they found that it was the appropriateness of the child's "*concept* of same and different," rather than perceptual ability or attentional factors, that made the crucial difference in letter reversals. More recently, Valett (1978) has reviewed the literature on teaching children to think and has illustrated several approaches to the development of mediational language skills in young children.

Studies on mediational thinking in children emphasize the importance of critical verbal concepts. Through the understanding and use of such concepts as "same and different," the child acquires internalized linguistic tools essential for problem solving. Reading and other learning beyond the first grade require the student to make increasingly difficult linguistic abstractions. For this reason it is important that children be taught mediational thinking strategies and helped to acquire key verbal concepts. For example, the Boehm Test of Basic Concepts (Boehm 1967) presents fifty basic verbal concepts in the three major categories of space ("middle," "over"), quantity ("most," "half"), and time ("never," "always") that a student should understand by the second grade. Dyslexic children need to be taught these basic verbal concepts systematically in order for any reading program to be effective.

Expressive Ability.   The expressive language abilities include all the many means of communicating thoughts, ideas, and feelings. Even body language belongs in this area, but spoken language with directed verbalization quickly becomes more important. An infant who is angry or in distress communicates through a combination of expressive body language and oral outbursts, but by the early school years, the child relies more on oral expressive language. Most kindergarten and first-grade children speak without difficulty, although articulation and syntax are still being developed.

However, dyslexic children often have a history of oral language deficiencies in the preschool years. In a summary of the neurological basis of reading disability, Martha Denckla (1977) of the Boston Children's Hospital Medical Center states that the following oral language deficiencies were the ones most frequently found in the early history of dyslexic children:

• naming and word-finding difficulties

- problems in remembering words

- poor memory for digits and sentences

- inaccurate articulation of speech sounds

- poor phonemic perception and sequencing of sounds

Denckla also found that boys distort names more than girls by confusing phonemes and through the inappropriate sequencing of sounds.

It should be apparent that children with receptive sensory-perceptual processing dysfunctions struggle to mediate, associate, and integrate sounds and to make some sense out of incomplete and distorted sensory data. The struggle results in distorted and delayed speech and interferes with other forms of expressive language.

Interrelated Abilities.   All language skills are interrelated and reinforce each other, so that no skill should be taught in complete isolation. Trying to teach reading to dyslexic children without also teaching listening, speaking, and writing interferes with their perception of linguistic relationships. Effective educational programs for dyslexic children take into account that speaking, reading, writing, and spelling are all dependent on interrelated auditory, visual, and kinesthetic functions.

One outstanding integrated language approach for teaching dyslexic children was devised by Anna Gillingham (Childs 1968), whose program will be discussed in detail later. Valett (1974) suggests another approach that arranges fifty-three learning abilities into skills and tasks. Six major categories emerge: gross-motor tasks, sensory-motor tasks, perceptual-motor (including auditory, visual, and visual-motor) tasks, conceptual skills, social skills, and language skills. Language skills are as follows: vocabulary, fluency and encoding, articulation, word-attack skills, reading comprehension, writing, and spelling. These skills and tasks are arranged in a hierarchy that considers the educational needs of dyslexic children. It is important to remember that no skill can be developed in a vacuum; as a child gains proficiency in one area, the way is paved for advancement in others.

The importance of interrelated language abilities is widely acknowledged by most authorities (Kirk, Kliebhan, and Lerner 1978) and is officially recognized by the U.S. Office of Education (1977, p. 65082):

Children with specific learning disabilities means those children who have a disorder in one or more of the basic psychological processes involved in *understanding or in using language, spoken or written* (emphasis mine), which disorder may manifest itself in imperfect ability to listen, think, speak, read, write, spell, or do mathematic calculations. Such disorders include such conditions as perceptual handicaps, brain injury, minimal brain dysfunction, dyslexia, and developmental aphasia. Such terms do not include children who have learning problems which are primarily the result of visual, hearing, or motor handicaps, or mental retardation, of emotional disturbance, or of environmental disadvantage.

Dyslexic children usually have a disorder in *more* than one of the basic psychological processes. These disorders interfere with their understanding and use of spoken *and* written language. Their receptive, mediational, and expressive language abilities are all impaired to some degree. However, since dyslexic children are frequently of average or better-than-average intelligence, it is possible for them to develop their language abilities and to learn to compensate for their disabilities. With special experience, training, and high motivation, many dyslexics, such as inventor Thomas Edison, brain surgeon Harvey Cushing, General George Patton, and former Vice President Nelson Rockefeller, have learned to use language skills and abilities to their advantage (Thompson 1971).

NORMAL DEVELOPMENTAL STAGES

Language abilities and stages of language development are interrelated, but to make discussion more convenient, we divide them here into seven developmental stages.

Stage 1: Sensory-Motor Exploration.

In the preverbal stage, the child explores, attends to, and acts on the environment. The essential element at this stage is exploratory play, which becomes the foundation for all later language and cognitive development (Bruner 1975). The work of Piaget (1951) shows that play is an indispensable step in stimulating the child's imagination and motivation for interacting with the world. During this exploratory stage the child begins to carry on an internal monologue during play. This monologue becomes the foundation for more formal operational thinking (Piaget and Inhelder 1969).

Stage 2: Babbling.   As the child moves about, plays, and interacts with the environment, he or she makes use of the vocalizations referred to as babbling. By the fifth or sixth month of life most children have begun to babble. By the age of twelve months these babbles begin to be self-reinforcing and develop into a rhythmic, patterned, nonsense speech complete with associated grunts, facial expressions, and gestures.

Studies by Conger, Kagan, and Mussen (1969) suggest that vocalizations can be increased in three-month-old infants if the mother rewards the child with smiles and touching. Mothers who vocalize to their babies stimulate vocal expression in them during the second half of their first year of life.

Stage 3: Imitation.   As children refine their vocalizations, they begin to imitate what they hear. *Echolalia* is imitative speech in which the child tries to echo what parents and others say. The child then experiments with the words in varied forms and patterns.

Research by Bricker and Bricker (1974) shows how early language training strategies that emphasize precommunication skills with much motor and verbal imitation help the child understand language. Adults should respond to a child's imitative speech with "cued language": question and comments that clarify and differentiate sounds for the child.

Stage 4: Differentiation.   After the early months of listening to and making sounds, a child begins to make specific associations with those sounds. They are then integrated into words that the child learns to recognize. By careful listening, and through imitative verbalization, the child learns that words can represent objects and feelings. Spoken language begins to emerge from the integration of images and ideas, and the child attempts to formulate and communicate experience.

The naming of objects, feelings, and experiences is a critical step in the differentiation of language. Beginning with single words, the child goes on to several words and begins to understand semantic and syntactical relationships. At three years old the child's language has a grammatical complexity resembling the language forms used by most adults (Dale 1976). The Conger, Kagan, and Mussen studies show that the average five-year-old has a vocabulary of over two thousand words and can construct complete sentences with correct grammatical organization. In the preschool years most of this language develops through imitation, modeling, and incidental learning.

Stage 5: Conceptualization. Through the process of naming, the child's vocabulary and verbal concepts develop further. A positive correlation exists between social exploration and involvement and the acquisition of words and language. Schiefelbusch, Copeland, and Smith (1967) describe in some detail how the acquisition of language is dependent upon the child's continual interaction with, and reinforcement from, the world. From such interactions the young child begins to classify and order the objects in the environment. Words are clasified and associated in meaningful syntactical order ("forks and spoons are to eat with"), and each acquired verbal concept in turn develops others.

The goals of early language development are outlined by Bloom and Lahey (1978). These authors stress that comprehension should be emphasized through teaching the "verbal content, form, and use" of words in beginning sentences. They also feel that if improved speech and comprehension do not follow repeated general language development sessions, prescriptively programmed lessons should be planned.

As part of her work in adapting Piaget's theories to early childhood education, Lavatelli (1970) devised a program for training children in language. In this approach, teachers use modeling and actions to elicit verbalizations while children engage in spontaneous self-directed activities. Lavatelli found that at this early stage of development "drill" instruction is not natural and defeats itself. Nevertheless, in small conversation groups, a warm, friendly, and supportive person can elicit fairly complex phrases from children.

Stage 6: Structural Generalization. As a child's thoughts and associations become more extended, his or her speech grows in complexity. Story language develops as the child gives structure to recalled or imagined experience: children organize stories into beginnings, middles, and ends and can recognize and paraphrase plots.

Structural generalization is an advanced stage during which expressive language ability is rapidly refined. Simple sentences are followed by more complex speech and the increasingly correct use of forms and expressions.

Most linguists recognize a physiological and biological basis for language and argue that there is an inherent human predisposition toward grammar in natural speech (Chomsky 1972). Structural generalizations that are the basis of grammatical rules emerge naturally in the developing language of young children and do not usually have to be formally taught.

It is true, though, that the child who is significantly delayed in structural generalization can and should be helped through early intervention and special forms of education. For example, Larsen (1974) found that structural teaching involving verbalization (naming, labeling, comparing, and so forth) and teacher demonstration helped children develop such concepts as classification, reversibility, coordination of attributes, and time, space, and quantity.

In an earlier study, Blank and Solomon (1968) devised an individual tutorial language program to develop abstract thinking in socially disadvantaged preschool children. In daily fifteen to twenty-minute training sessions over a four-month period, children were taught to pay attention to, categorize, and verbalize cause and effect relations. These sessions resulted in significant improvement in language ability and a fourteen-point rise in IQ scores.

In a similar study, Bernstein (1970) divided eighty kindergarten children (who had failed language pretests) into an experimental and a control group. The experimental group was asked to solve object problems and discuss the similarities of objects in a particular group. They were also asked to contrast objects in one group with those in another group. Significant advances in language were found in the experimental group over the controls following training, and these advances were retained by the children in later tests.

Stage 7: Symbolic-Operational Control.

This is the final stage of language development, and most children do not reach it until about eleven years of age. By this age a person demonstrates abilities—thoughtful speech, verbal fluency, representational drawing, silent and oral reading, spelling, and writing—that arise in the language centers of the brain.

These forms of expressive language are shaped by the child's formal education. During the primary and elementary school years, interest, motivation, and the refinement of specific language skills are essential elements in the development of advanced symbolic operations. There are many contributing factors to success during the formative primary school years.

One excellent teaching model for use in transitional preschool-primary instruction was designed by Bellugi-Klima and Hass (1968). In this model, the teacher carefully notes the immature syntactical structure the child uses. Then he or she models the correct syntax and encourages the child to repeat it by asking a question that demands the use of that structure in response. Some examples of the recommended developmental instructional sequence presented in this model are as follows:

Plurals

The *beads* are in the box.

Simple Past

Yesterday we *played* with the beads.

Prepositions

Put the beads *behind* the triangle.

Modal True/False Statements

The beads *can't* be put in the same group with the cars.

Affirmative Questions

Are these beads red?

Negative Questions

Isn't this bead square?

"Wh" (Who, What, Where, When, Which, Why) Questions

What can you use these beads for?

Coordinations

Put the beads *and* the blocks in the yellow box.

Comparatives

Point to the one that is *longer* and *thinner*.

Temporal Connectives

Raise your hand *after* you have placed the beads on the string.

Most children learn symbolic-operational language in family settings. Milner (1951) conducted a study of the relationship between reading readiness in first-grade children and the patterns of parent-child interactions. He found that families of children who achieved high scores on language test items ate together and conversed during meals. In the families of children with low scores, children ate separately or the group did not converse.

One of the most widely used models for teaching basic language operations to young disadvantaged children was designed by Bereiter and Engelmann (1966). This is a five-step approach:

Step 1—Repetition
Teacher (T): This is a red apple.
Student (S): This is a red apple.

Step 2—Yes/No Questions
T: Is this apple green?
S: No, that apple is not green.

Step 3—Location Tasks
T: Show me an apple that is red.
S: This apple is red.

Step 4—Making Statements
T: Tell me about this apple.
S: This apple is round, shiny, red . . . .
T: Tell me what this apple is not.
S: This apple is not green. It is not square. It is not dirty.

Step 5—Deduction Problems
T: (With hidden apple) This apple is not red. Do you know what color it is?
S: No, it might be green or yellow . . . .

NEUROPSYCHOLOGICAL CORRELATES

Masland (1967) gives a detailed explanation of brain mechanisms and their correlation to language. Using schematic drawings, Masland identifies the brain areas in which language is mediated and suggests how established language forms may break down with brain impairment. Citing the work of Kornoski, Masland explains how, through babbling, the child learns to associate certain sounds with certain movements of the mouth and tongue. Babbling thus creates and strengthens neural paths in the auditory areas of the brain. This is one of the first neuropsychological steps in language development. Then, by mimicking, the child reinforces neural integration of sound, sensation, and movement and prepares for the development of associative meaning.

In most persons, language functions are developed in the left hemisphere of the brain. But there are exceptions, as, for instance, those who have received a serious injury to the left side of the brain before they reach the age of eight. "In such individuals it is well established that adequate language functions can be subserved by the right hemisphere" (Masland, p. 5). Receptive language disorders result from a variety of cortical auditory imperceptions (sometimes referred to as "central deafness") that interfere with the primary auditory cortex process of making proper auditory discrimination or forming correct associations.

Reading is basically a neuropsychological process of making discriminative responses to graphic symbols. Many neurologists, such as Gomez (1971) and others, say that responses are dependent on the earlier acquisition of neural processing abilities to attend to sounds, to decode and associate sounds, and to program the auditory cortex.

Vellutino (1977) suggests that dyslexia and other severe reading disabilities seem to be disorders in one or more aspects of psycholinguistic functioning, such as in the semantic, syntactic, and phonological components of language. Many of these linguistic disorders, especially those in young boys, are correlated to a great degree with maturational delays. For example, Satz (1976) conducted a number of dichotic listening experiments with five- to twelve-year-old reading-disabled children and a group of nondisabled controls. He found that good readers have a right ear advantage (REA) at all ages studied and that the magnitude of the advantage increases with age. By contrast, the results with dyslexic children reveal a lag in the development of ear asymmetry with no great REA at any age (although a right-ear *preference* does exist from the age of seven).

Other evidence shows that dyslexic children have reading difficulties because their brains mature more slowly or are deficient in the anatomical connections needed to learn reading in the usual ways (Gardner 1973). Studies by Nemac (1978) on hemiplegics demonstrate that patients with left-hemisphere damage were significantly more distractible while performing a verbal task with verbal interference than those with right-hemisphere damage. There were similar results in tests of vision.

Farr (1969) reports that retarded readers tend to score higher on the WISC Performance Scale than on the Verbal Scale. Poor readers score lowest on Information, Arithmetic, Digit Span, and Coding subtests. Searls (1975) and Griffiths (1977) discuss the use of the WISC as a diagnostic-remedial tool for dyslexia. In a similar study on the influence of cerebral lesions on psychological test performance of older children, Reed, Reitan, and Kløve (1965) found significant test patterns: these investigators compared fifty brain-damaged children with fifty uninjured children (all ten to fourteen years old). Subtests of the Halstead-Reitan Neuropsychological Battery and the Wechsler Intelligence Scale for Children were administered to all subjects. The uninjured children significantly exceeded those with brain damage on all subtests. The single most discriminating Wechsler subtest was the Digit Symbol memory test where 82 percent of the uninjured children achieved higher scores than the neurologically impaired group.

All these studies demonstrate that dyslexia is a complex neuro-psychological syndrome of associated linguistic disorders. These language dysfunctions cannot be cleanly separated. They demand a team approach for evaluation, developmental education, and remediation.

LANGUAGE DISORDERS IN CHILDREN

Tasks that evaluate auditory-perceptual integration are the best means to discover language disorders in children. Sabatino (1969) used the pairing of nonsense syllables to identify neurologically impaired children. He also tested with tasks such as meaningful word discrimination, immediate recall of digits, memory for sentences, duplication of tapped rhythms, and comprehension of simple stories. All of these tests tap central auditory processing functions essential in most forms of expressive language. Because of complex neuro-psychological interrelationships, it is impossible to state that one form of a language disorder exists by itself. However, the segregation of these disorders into academic categories and the use of certain accepted definitions can prove useful in diagnosis and in planning remedial strategies:

Receptive Language Dysfunction. A dysfunction in the sensory-perceptual channels and the central nervous system. It blocks or distorts the integration of sensory stimuli and impairs both comprehension and expression. Severe auditory problems interfere with attending, listening, following directions, and learning.

Dysarthria. A severe motor problem of the jaw and tongue resulting from central nervous system damage. Speech is slurred and frequently unintelligible. Commonly seen in children with cerebral palsy. Except in very rare cases, loss of speech is accompanied by other language disturbances, such as the inability to associate motor patterns and speech sounds. A detailed clinical study of delayed language in such a child (with a discussion of psychological test correlates) has been published by Taylor (1961).

Developmental Dysphasia.   A severe delay in the acquisition of speech and expressive language due to neuropsychological problems. These children have a slow rate of language acquisition (approximately half that of normal elementary-school children). Eisenson and Ingram (1972) summarize the specific language deficiencies as inability or delay in:

- organizing sensory-auditory events
- retaining or holding events in mind
- scanning events and comparing them with others
- using sentences and speech inflections and deriving meaning from words

This disorder is also commonly referred to as *developmental aphasia* although this term is technically incorrect if there is no evidence of *loss* of language.

Aphasia.   This term refers to language impairment *after* language has been acquired in the normal manner. The major causes are tumors; infectious diseases, such as meningitis; degenerative diseases, such as multiple sclerosis; and traumatic brain accidents, such as those incurred in automobile crashes, poisoning, and so forth. The most common language difficulty of aphasics is their inability to speak correctly due to decoding, memory, and syntax problems (Schuell 1974). Because aphasics are easily frustrated, Osgood (1963) stresses the importance of relaxation, play, pantomime, and high motivational activities along with intensive auditory training.

Dyslexia.   A congenital developmental delay or impairment in the ability to translate sounds into letter symbols and to comprehend written material. Most authorities, such as Keeney and Keeney (1966), stress that the major impairment is not in recognition or discrimination but rather in symbol interpretation. Dyslexic children almost always have several language problems that result in significantly poor reading performance.

Dysgraphia.   Significant developmental disability or impairment in writing. Usually evidenced in extremely poor letter formations, disorganization, and limited fine visual-motor coordination. Success in remediating these problems correlates with the overall development of language skills emphasizing directional, temporal, and spatial concept training and anxiety reduction (Laurita 1971).

Alexia.   The *loss* of established ability to read. Usually accompanied by some loss of writing skills (agraphia). The person can, however, speak and understand spoken language.

One of the most famous cases was described in 1891 by the French neurologist Joseph Jules Dejerine and recently discussed by Geschwind (1972). Postmortem examination of this patient showed a lesion in the angular gyrus of the left hemisphere and in the splenium section of the corpus callosum. Although the subject saw words and letters correctly, they were meaningless to him. He was unable to match what he saw with a corresponding sound pattern. "Patients suffering from alexia with agraphia cannot recognize words spelled aloud to them nor can they spell aloud a spoken word" (Geschwind 1972, p. 83).

Geschwind's work shows that children recover from cerebral damage more completely than adults, which fact supports the view that in childhood the right hemisphere does have some capacity to take over speech functions from a damaged left hemisphere.

Orton (1964) states that the cause of all the foregoing disabilities in childhood is very closely related to physiological dysfunction within the brain. Orton also describes the most common characteristic in all of these disorders as a difficulty in making the correct sequence of letters, sounds, or movements. He recommends that remedial training begin with simple blending exercises consisting of only one consonant followed by one vowel. Then, when this simple process is mastered, more extensive and demanding auditory-vocal sequences should be introduced.

Developmental-remedial treatment for language disorders is a complex undertaking that requires team effort. There are many possible treatment approaches; these are described in detail by Wood (1964), Lahey (1978), and others. Some of the more important members of this team, and their major role in language development or treatment, are listed below.

Parents.   Parents are the primary observers of their children. Their critical role is carefully observing and reporting language behaviors and supporting, reinforcing, and motivating their children as they develop language abilities. Public Law 94-142 (the "Education for All Handicapped Children" Act) requires consultation with and involvement of parents in the planning of individual educational programs for their children, including discussion of instructional goals and objectives.

Regular Classroom Teachers.   Since federal law now requires that dyslexic and other exceptional children be educated in the "least restrictive environment," all regular teachers are involved. In most classrooms emphasis is placed on the development of basic language and reading skills. As a member of the team working with dyslexic children, the regular teacher helps to individualize and modify the regular program and cooperates with parents and special educators in reinforcing and supplementing prescriptive instruction.

Special Educator.   Most dyslexic children will require special education from a specialist in learning disabilities. This person coordinates the diagnostic-prescriptive efforts in the local school, provides unique neuropsychological education using lessons, materials, and equipment not available in regular classrooms, and serves as a central resource person to other team members.

Speech and Language Specialist.   The dyslexic child with significantly delayed speech and related language disorders such as faulty articulation, hesitant speech (stuttering, stammering), voice problems, and other forms of expressive difficulties, will undoubtedly require evaluation and remedial services from a speech and language specialist. In many programs these specialists also work closely with both regular and special educators in helping them to design and follow programs of auditory training and systematic language acquisition as well as other forms of diagnostic-prescriptive language instruction.

Reading Teachers.   In most schools, teachers who are especially well trained in reading instruction are assigned time for remedial reading. Usually, these teachers work in reading-resource centers or reading clinics that provide instruction both individually and in small groups. Such reading centers are supplied with language development materials that permit children to be placed and programmed at their own levels and to progress at their own rates.

School Psychologist.   The major role of the psychologist is to serve as a consultant to other team members in helping them devise, carry through, and evaluate the diagnostic-prescriptive program. The psychologist often administers special tests and serves as a liaison with physicians and other specialists. Many psychologists also provide parent counseling and educational programs that increase cooperation between home and school.

Physician.   All dyslexic children require medical evaluation and supervision. The prompt diagnosis and treatment of early childhood diseases is extremely important. Physicians give guidance in obtaining auditory training and proper medical treatment, in learning sound nutritional habits, and in maintaining good health.

School Administrators.   The school principal must always be involved as a key team member in any special program. Parents must usually take the initiave in seeing and conferring with new principals and other important administrators, such as coordinators or directors of special education programs.

DEVELOPMENTAL-REMEDIAL LANGUAGE APPROACHES

Numerous programs have been created to develop receptive, mediational, and expressive language abilities. In this final section we will summarize some of them.

Preschool Programs.   Bereiter and Engelmann (1966) were among the first to show that special cognitive training in verbal skills for disadvantaged preschool children stimulated intellectual growth and resulted in significant linguistic and mental improvement. Blank and Solomon (1968) conducted a study with preschool children that has been used as a model for more recent programs.

Klaus and Gray (1968) made a five-year follow-up on disadvantaged three-year-olds who had been involved in a program teaching classification, generalization, and expanded syntax. For example, the children were taught the word "trike." Then they were instructed and rewarded for saying "Could I please have the trike?" Finally they were taught complex sentence structure, such as "Could I have the tricycle that John is using when he is through?" These children gained nine IQ points over control children and the gains persisted into the primary grades.

A study by Brainerd (1974) with 144 preschool children divided into 72 experimental and 72 control subjects shows that specific verbal concepts can be taught systematically at this early age. By means of verbal feedback and discussion contingent upon correct response, these children made significant improvement in the development of selected verbal concepts such as conservation (weight and volume remain as constants in the child's mind during observed physical changes of state).

The most extensive study of this kind was conducted by Heber (1972, 1976) and his colleagues at the University of Wisconsin. This group created a detailed cognitive-language orientation curriculum for preschool children using planned environmental stimulation and prescriptive teaching with several major language components. Language instruction was carried out as part of the program referred to as the "Milwaukee Project." This preschool language curriculum included lessons in comprehension, vocabulary acquisition, communication, and critical thinking (such as guessing games and prediction of outcomes). The preschool reading program included readiness lessons in the acquisition of visual and auditory skills and in alphabet recognition and discrimination. This preschool program was followed by a more formal reading program emphasizing language experience approaches, but also including introductory phonics.

In the Milwaukee Project the Illinois Test of Psycholinguistic Abilities (ITPA) was used as a criterion instrument. The ITPA was administered to all children at the age of four and a half and again at six and a half. At six and a half the experimental group performed at six months above their chronological age while the control group was eleven months below chronological age. As a result of special language training, the experimental group developed an average psycholinguistic quotient of 108.3 (22 points over the control group). Other criterion tests and measures confirmed the significant language development of the experimental group. Extensive follow-up studies show that these language gains persisted through the primary school years and contributed to academic success in reading.

Many other preschool studies show that the acquisition of basic language skills can be significantly boosted in the early preschool years through the use of concentrated instruction. Appropriate prescriptive instruction in the preschool years can contribute to a gain in language and reading readiness scores of six months or more, which gain may prove critical for some dyslexic children.

Early Childhood and Primary School Years.   Several years ago Lovaas, Berberich, Perloff, and Schaeffer (1966) designed a successful program to help young schizophrenic children acquire imitative speech. These children were gradually taught words and language using verbal discrimination training with food as a reinforcement.

Another successful imitative modeling strategy for instructing language-disordered children five to ten years old was devised by Courtright and Courtright (1976). They found that exposing the children to correct language patterns and having them subvocalize what they heard was more effective than trying to teach specific rules of speech. In a similar study, Ammon and Ammon (1971) trained young black children in specific vocabulary and in elaborative sentence constructions. They found that their experimental group showed significant improvement in vocabulary acquisition but *not* in sentence construction, and they recommend that early training should emphasize vocabulary development.

Most language training programs for slow learners and the retarded stress the importance of acquiring receptive and expressive visual-auditory skills and basic vocabulary (Darnell and Molineux 1972). A systematic study of vocabulary development in 107 mentally retarded children from eight to eleven years old was conducted by Taylor, Thurlow, and Turnure (1977). The children received fifteen vocabulary lessons, each containing five new words. All words were presented in stories about money, time, and airplanes. Test results showed that students who learned new vocabulary words in integrated projects using pictorial material and tape recordings used the newly acquired words and themes in their own conversations. The researchers recommend that selected concrete words be taught first and the more abstract multiple-meaning words be introduced later.

A number of relatively new techniques have also been developed to stimulate language in handicapped children. De Pauw (1978) worked with aphasic children who demonstrated severe disability in either the comprehension or expression of language. These children were given twenty minutes of sensory-motor training daily for seven months. Significant gains were made over controls on four subtests of the Southern California Sensory Integration Test, and it was also noted (but not conclusively) that spontaneous language appeared to increase both during and after sensory-motor training activities.

Years ago Kohl (1966) advocated that sign language be given greater emphasis with young deaf and hearing-impaired children. He argued that sign language could be used to stimulate oral expressiveness and to show the child why oral language has advantages. The Seattle Public Schools actually devised and implemented a total communication program with handicapped students from three to twenty-one years old. Words were presented by both name and signs with resulting improvement in articulation. Many parents reported that this program produced the first real communication they had ever experienced with their children (Grinnell, Detamore, and Lippke 1976).

Other forms of sign-symbol language have also proved successful with language-disordered children. DeVilliers and Naughton (1974) used a "particle language" consisting of English words and signs printed on magnetic particles and arranged on a magnetic board. Autistic children were taught simple syntax, comprehension, and simple commands and questions by this method.

For profoundly verbally handicapped persons, electronic workboards have been created. One such example is the "Form-A-Phrase" board (see Appendix). The board is devised so that the impaired person can control sound units to express common words and sentences. Controls are manipulated by hand, headpointers, or mouthsticks.

Many successful language development methods, materials, and techniques have been integrated into special curriculums and classes. There is a trend toward early placement of language-disabled children in developmental programs where concentrated team instruction and effort can be coordinated. Several successful models for such classes are now available.

One of these models is discussed in great detail by Monaco and Zaslow (1972) and grew out of extensive applied research with a class for children with severe language disabilities in the Montgomery County, Maryland, public schools. In this model emphasis is placed on initial diagnostic assessment and closely related remedial instruction. Monaco and Zaslow also present an excellent case study of a boy ("Timmy") that illustrates in detail how severe language disabilities relate to reading and academic performance problems and how such a child was given special education.

Middle Elementary School Years.   During the middle elementary grades, concrete language is gradually transformed to representational and preoperational symbolic forms. Expressive language becomes more formally shaped with increasing emphasis placed on fluency and correctness in oral reading, writing, and spelling. Most school workbooks and instructional materials are of this more demanding, abstract type. But even at this relatively advanced level, many special approaches can be used to facilitate language learning.

Enstrom and Enstrom (1969) argue that the elimination of writing reversals such as *b–d* confusion, strengthens reading performance by eliminating letter distortion and thereby furthers integration during the formal reading process.

Such varied techniques as the use of comic strips and medication have also been used to improve writing skills. Hallenbeck (1976) devised a series of comic strips and tape-recorded stories to develop language sequencing, left-right progression, discrimination of details, abstract thinking, and correlated writing abilities. Other studies, such as the recent one by Arnold, Huestis, Wemmer, and Smeltzer (1978), demonstrate the value of using appropriate stimulant drugs (such as dextroamphetamine) to improve visual-motor performance in the drawing and writing of children with minimal brain dysfunction.

Spelling is an advanced language ability that particularly frustrates dyslexic children. John Arena (1968) has collated a number of successful approaches to building spelling skills in dyslexic persons. Among the best techniques is that of having the student dictate his or her own spelling list on tape by both pronouncing and spelling the word. The child then plays back the list of five to ten words, writes the words while listening to them, and corrects the spelling by relistening to the tape. Spelling is the translation of perceived sounds into letter names (oral spelling) and into letter forms (written spelling). The Gillingham and Stillman (1960) program of remedial training for children with specific disability in reading, spelling, and penmanship is an integrated approach to total language development that is highly recommended.

SUMMARY   Dyslexic children are usually deficient in the acquisition and development of several language abilities. Receptive language, mediational-associative language, and expressive language are the major abilities these children are deficient in. All of these abilities are interrelated and nonseparable.

Children progress through stages of language acquisition and development. These stages include sensory-motor exploration, babbling, imitation, differentiation, conceptualization, structural generalization, and symbolic-operational control. There are neuropsychological correlates that occur for each psycholinguistic process. Disorders in these processes may result in receptive language dysfunction, dysarthia, developmental dysphasia, aphasia, dyslexia, dysgraphia, alexia, and other interrelated language problems requiring a team approach for diagnosis and remediation.

A number of approaches to the acquisition and development of language skills and abilities have emerged from research and practice. Giordano (1978) reviews research on language development, linguistics, neuropsychology, and its implications for teaching reading and concludes that reading should be taught as a communicative language skill. Reading instruction should begin with a representative inventory of the child's vocabulary, semantics, and syntax. All lessons should be structured to aid the child to understand what results are expected. Instruction in reading should use two or more modalities (hearing, speech, silent reading, writing, and others) in every lesson, and these lessons should be designed to transfer to oral forms of communication.

Some of the distinctive characteristics of selected preschool, primary, and middle-elementary-school programs were reviewed. For dyslexic children with associated language disabilities, a recommended instructional strategy is to:

1. make a tape-recorded sample of the child's expressive language

2. transcribe the child's vocabulary, meaning, and sentence structure

3. select specific words to be taught and used in subsequent developmental language lessons

4. list the language objectives to be demonstrated in terms of number of words, sentence length, meaning, and so forth

5. design the instructional program using multisensory interrelated language forms

6. systematically reinforce the child at home and at school for specific language acquisition

7. let the children initiate spontaneous language-building activities

8. make sure the child understands and uses his or her newly acquired language in meaningful forms of communication

In a review of many studies on the development of receptive and expressive language in handicapped children, Snyder, Lovitt, and Smith (1975) conclude that it is possible to improve language skills through instructional techniques and reinforcement strategies. The language abilities of dyslexic children can be developed and their disabilities can be remediated or compensated for through appropriate forms of special education.

DISCUSSION QUESTIONS AND ACTIVITIES

1. What is receptive language?

2. Describe some of the cognitive operations required in using mediational-associative language.

3. How can teachers find out what verbal concepts a first-grade child might possess?

4. List some of the oral-language deficiencies most frequently found in young dyslexic children.

5. What are some of the major forms of expressive language?

6. How can infant vocalizations and babbling be increased?

7. Discuss the critical steps in the differentiation stage of language acquisition.

8. How does the young child develop grammar? How well is grammar acquired by the time the average child starts public school?

9. Discuss the implications of Bernstein's (1970) experimental study.

10. Discuss the Bellugi-Klima/Hass model of language acquisition.

11. At what stage of language acquisition may the Bereiter-Engelmann model be helpful?

12. What are the implications of Satz's (1976) study on dichotic listening?

13. Define *dyslexia*.

14. How might a special educator use the findings of Sabatino's study on evaluating auditory-perceptual integration?

15. Discuss the similarities and differences between dysphasia/aphasia, and dyslexia/alexia.

16. What may happen to a person when a lesion develops in the splenium section of the corpus callosum?

17. What did Samuel Orton recommend as the beginning point in developmental-remedial language training?

18. Discuss the role of several members of the diagnostic-prescriptive team involved in the treatment or education of dyslexic children.

19. Review current reports on Heber's Milwaukee Project and discuss the results.

20. Summarize some of the research regarding developmental-remedial language instruction for handicapped children.

21. Use the recommended eight-step instructional strategy on page 58 for designing, teaching, and reporting on a language lesson for a dyslexic child.

CHAPTER FIVE

Diagnosis

We have defined dyslexia as a significant disorder in the meaningful integration of perceptual-linguistic symbols due to neuropsychological immaturity or dysfunction. In preschool children of normal intelligence the disorder usually appears in the gross immaturity of psycholinguistic abilities and reading-readiness skills. In school-age children of normal intelligence a lag of two or more years in functional reading and associated perceptual-linguistic skills is usually symptomatic of the disorder.

With this pragmatic definition we can proceed with the operational steps involved in the diagnosis of dyslexia. Differential diagnosis is important if we assume that dyslexic children need and profit from specific forms of treatment and remediation. The unique behavioral manifestations of this disorder are summarized by many investigators such as George Spache (1976) and include:

- disorganization, reversals, and "twisting" of symbols
- dysfunction in auditory/visual sequential memory
- problems in the rhythmic patterning of sounds, rhymes, words, and sentences
- difficulty in sustaining focused attention

61

- disorders in body organization, coordination, and sensory integration
- associated copying, writing, and drawing distortions

The diagnostic problem is to determine how well the person is reading, what fundamental reading skills are missing or undeveloped, to what extent dyslexic behaviors are demonstrated, and whether or not these can reasonably be attributed to neuropsychological dysfunction or immaturity. As Rabinovitch (1959) emphasizes, dyslexia is a disability that is symptomatic of a biological weakness in integrating symbolic written material. The determination of psychoneurological and biological inadequacies is largely a clinical process of qualitative and quantitative evaluation that is seldom done effectively.

Proper diagnosis requires the professional assessment of the child's reading performance and related abilities. A summary of the diagnostic steps advocated by Kirk (1962) and Rabinovitch (1959), among others, follows:

Determine Functional Reading Level.   Functional reading level is reflected in the kinds of reading material understood with ease.

Determine Reading Potential and Capacity.   Potential or capacity is reflected in differential achievement on varied reading and psycholinguistic tasks including tests of general mental ability.

Determine Extent of Reading Disability.   A significant disability exists if the child's functional reading level is two or more years behind his or her potential.

Determine Specific Reading Skill Deficiencies.   Deficiencies are determined through a task analysis of the student's functional reading and by a detailed analysis of psychoeducational test results.

Determine Neuropsychological Dysfunction.   Neuropsychological dysfunction is reflected in the pattern and quality of test results and by the clinical appraisal of selected behavior such as attention span, body organization, and sensory integration.

Determine Associated Factors.   Associated factors in primary reading disorders include the lack of motivation, interest, or reinforcement; anxiety or fear of reading; inadequate instruction or opportunity to learn to read; and gross sensory impairment or ill health.

Determine Developmental-Remedial Strategies. Meaningful strategies must include the specification of the main learning objectives and of tasks for improving neuropsychological processing and integration of perceptual-linguistic skills.

Proper diagnosis requires the cooperation of the classroom teacher, special educator, psychologist, and physician. However, the major part of the diagnostic evaluation should be done by the special educator in cooperation with the referring teacher since they will be primarily responsible for the implementation of diagnostic objectives. Below we elaborate on each of these diagnostic steps.

DETERMINING FUNCTIONAL READING LEVEL

Most reading is done silently although it is sometimes necessary to read aloud in delivering a report or speech. The essential thing to be considered is comprehension, or the meaningfulness of the material to the person who is reading. This is best determined through a direct assessment of both oral and silent reading.

Spache (1976, p. 314) suggests testing the child in both oral and silent reading using the basal readers assigned in his or her grade. The child is working at grade level when he or she can read one hundred words with *at least 70 percent comprehension* and with no more than twenty technical or mechanical errors, such as phonetic mistakes, omissions, or distortions. Since all schools have a developmental series of basal readers available, teachers can easily determine any child's functional reading level.

In addition to the direct assessment of reading in the classroom, some standardized reading tests should be used. For determining functional performance and achievement, both group and individually administered tests must be used. Although tests vary considerably, all good reading tests include a number of items that measure fundamental psycholinguistic reading skills and abilities. Some of the more critical perceptual-linguistic skills required in learning to read that are commonly included in tests are listed in Table 4.

Below are examples of three group reading tests.

The Comprehensive Tests of Basic Skills—Level A (CTB/McGraw-Hill Division) is illustrative of a good reading-readiness test that covers most of the critical perceptual-linguistic skills on the beginning level. It is given to kindergarten and early first-grade children and measures the following seven readiness skills:

1. Visual discrimination: choosing words or shapes that match a visual stimulus

2. Listening for information: matching pictures with vocabulary and verbal concepts

3. Letter forms: matching capital letters with the same lowercase letters

4. Letter names: selecting letters named aloud by the teacher from four choices

5. Letter sounds: identification of consonant and long and short vowel sounds

6. Sound matching: identifying whether words read aloud are the same as those on the test

7. Language: identifying whether sentences read aloud by the teacher are correctly or incorrectly phrased

TABLE 4. Critical Perceptual-Linguistic Skills

Visual Skills	Auditory Skills	Auditory-Visual-Verbal Integration	Kinesthetic Symbolization
Following picture-story sequences	Matching words and objects	Following simple directions	Matching objects and shapes
Matching identical pictures	Identifying rhyming words	Verbalizing story sequences	Matching different-sized letters
Matching identical letters and words	Discriminating initial consonants	Duplicating rhythmic patterns	Matching upper and lower case letters
Tracking letters in a sentence	Discriminating medial consonants	Repeating letter sequences	Copying letters and symbols
Tracking words in a sentence and paragraph	Discriminating final consonants	Repeating letter sounds, blends, syllables	Writing letters and symbols from dictation
Finding syllables and selected words	Discriminating vowel sounds	Repeating word sequences	Writing initial and final sounds
Locating paragraphs, headings, chapters	Discriminating blends	Verbally completing incomplete sentences with context words	Writing dictated vowels
	Discriminating syllables		Copying words
Visual closure and identification of partial or incomplete pictures, letters, words			Writing blends and syllables
			Writing dictated words

The Metropolitan Achievement Test—Primary I (Harcourt Brace Jovanovich) is a simple one-hour, three-part reading test for use in grades 1.5 to 2.4:

1. Word knowledge: Children look at a picture of a common object and must select from among four words the one that describes the picture.

2. Word analysis: Children identify a dictated word from among several words with similar configurations and sound patterns. For example: *tap* — tag / tape / tap / tab

3. Reading comprehension: Children read three simple sentences and mark the one that best describes a picture. They then read simple story paragraphs and mark the best summary sentence for each from a choice of several sentences.

The Stanford Diagnostic Reading Test—Level 1 (Harcourt Brace Jovanovich) is a more difficult and detailed diagnostic test for children from grades 2.5 to 4.5. It is a seven-part two-hour test, which must be given in sections. It evaluates higher cognitive functions, such as the comprehension of abstractions, as well as reading level.

1. Reading comprehension. Two- and three-sentence paragraphs are followed by multiple-choice answers requiring both understanding of content and inferential thinking. (30 minutes)

    Example: The camel lives in the desert.
    He has two big _____ on his back.
    ☐ babies ■ humps ☐ cups ☐ sacks

2. Auditory vocabulary. The child listens to a sentence read by the teacher and then marks the best response from three possible answers. (20 minutes)

    Example: A mother is a _____ .
    ☐ man ■ woman ☐ child

3. Auditory discrimination. The child listens to two words read by the teacher and then crosses out a *B* if the words begin the same, an *E* if they end the same or an *M* if the middle sound is the same. (20 minutes)

    Example: cake—make
    B ✗ (or) ✗

4. Syllabication. The child looks at a word and marks the first syllable from among three choices. (12 minutes)

   Example: baby
   ■ ba   ☐ bab   ☐ bay

5. Beginning and ending sounds. Pictures of common objects are presented with directions to mark either the beginning or ending sound of their names. (20 minutes)

   Example:

   ☐ m   ■ t   ☐ f   ☐ d

6. Blending. This is essentially a spelling test, which requires the child to divide dictated words in meaningful ways and then to synthesize and blend the sounds. (20 minutes)

   Example: Bird
   ☐ r   ■ ir   ■ d
   ■ b   ☐ a   ☐ n

7. Sound discrimination. The child reads a word, discriminates the sound underlined, then marks a word that has the same sound.

   Example: Like
   ☐ will   ☐ it   ■ ride

Each of the above tests is usually administered to a whole class or to small groups. Since group directions, time limitations, and other demands usually create stress and confusion and thus distract learning-disabled children, their group test results are highly unreliable. However the items on the test usually reflect actual classroom and curricular demands. For this reason, it is very important for the special educator to make a careful item analysis of these tests and then readminister parts of the test or the entire test if necessary (Brueckner and Bond 1955). Most group tests, such as the Stanford Diagnostic Reading Test, have much to offer in the way of diagnostic-prescriptive objectives if they are individually readministered and carefully interpreted.

It is always necessary to supplement data obtained from classroom observation and testing with individual psychoeducational appraisal. There are many good individual diagnostic reading tests. Those listed below are illustrative.

Gray Oral Reading Test (Bobbs Merrill Company) consists of a series of twelve developmental reading paragraphs.

Wide Range Reading and Spelling Tests (Guidance Associates) are two short and popular tests. The reading test measures sight vocabulary and must be supplemented with other comprehension and phonics tests.

The Larsen-Hammill Test of Written Spelling (Academic Therapy Publications) is a relatively new test. It helps determine the child's ability to spell both phonetically based and nonphonetic words with scores given in both spelling ages and grade equivalents.

Spache Diagnostic Reading Scales (California Test Bureau) is a good clinical test of reading vocabulary, comprehension, and basic phonetic skills including vowels, blends, and syllables.

DETERMINING READING POTENTIAL AND CAPACITY

A child often will perform better on an individual reading test than on a group test. Learning-disabled students also perform better on non-timed tests and tests given in sections to allow for movement and rest. Such differences reflect unused potential for learning to read.

Again, some children who do poorly on decoding written reading material demonstrate normal or superior comprehension when they are required to interpret stories and answer exact content questions after the story is read aloud. Or, the child who demonstrates a knowledge of most phonetic skills but lacks speed and efficiency might be judged to have good potential to learn syllabication and phrase reading if he or she receives special training.

In general, test results that approach or even surpass the normal range indicate a capacity for language learning despite poor performance at school. In the dyslexic child most parents and teachers recognize this differential performance and see an undeveloped potential. But learning potential must be quantified through a direct psychometric assessment of related verbal and performance abilities. Most schools administer group aptitude or scholastic-ability tests that require reading and differential problem solving. If the child can read and perform better on these tests (or parts of these tests) than in class, then he or she probably has the capacity to improve with more appropriate education.

But as we have already discusssed, group tests of achievement, aptitude, or ability are highly unreliable and must be supplemented with individual psychometric and clinical evaluation. Most regular teachers do not have the training or the time to administer individual psychometric tests. Individual ability, aptitude, and mental testing should be done by qualified diagnostic-prescriptive special educators and psychologists who can properly interpret this kind of test information. The tests listed below are a sample of those used by special educators to help determine reading potential and capacity.

The Peabody Picture Vocabulary Test (American Guidance Service) is a simple and direct test of a child's receptive language. A series of four pictures is presented, and the child must point to the picture named by the examiner. Mental age, percentiles, and intelligence quotient scores can be determined for children from two to seventeen years old. The mental age score here is really a receptive language age score and the resulting IQ is much more reliably interpreted as a receptive language quotient (RLQ). This is a good and helpful instrument to aid in determining language capacity and potential.

The Valett Developmental Survey of Basic Learning Abilities (Consulting Psychologists Press) consists of 233 tasks for children two through seven years old. Subtests include motor integration and physical development, tactile discrimination, auditory discrimination, visual-motor coordination, visual discrimination, language development and verbal fluency, and conceptual development. This test has been widely used by preschool and kindergarten specialists in the evaluation and programming of skills found to be prerequisite to formal reading.

The Wechsler Intelligence Scale for Children (Psychological Corporation) is generally administered by a psychologist who reports results to the teacher and special educator. They in turn interpret and integrate the findings with all other available information. The prescriptive use and interpretation of WISC scores are presented in detail by Glasser and Zimmerman (1967), Ferinden and Jacobson (1969), Wechsler (1974), and Valett (1978). One publication by Searls (1975) was sponsored by the International Reading Association and relates each subtest to the reading process. It is important to note that the WISC consists of two major scales. The Verbal Scale includes the six subtests of Information, Similarities, Arithmetic, Vocabulary, Comprehension, and Digit Span. The Performance Scale consists of six more subtests of Picture Completion, Picture Arrangement, Block Design, Object Assembly, Coding, and Mazes. From an analysis of subtest patterns and scores, the experienced clinician is able to deduce much about intellectual potential.

DETERMINING EXTENT OF READING DISABILITY

The determination of significant reading disability is a professional judgment of the discrepancy between the child's functional reading level and his or her reading potential or capacity. Such a judgment must take into consideration such related factors as chronological age, mental age and intelligence, grade-level placement, and current reading-achievement-test scores.

TABLE 5. Mental Age and Reading Grade Level Expectancies

Mental age	Reading grade expectancy	Mental age	Reading grade expectancy
6–2	1.0	10–4	5.0
6–5	1.3	10–8	5.3
6–8	1.5	10–11	5.5
7–0	1.8	11–2	5.8
7–2	2.0	11–5	6.0
7–6	2.3	11–8	6.3
7–8	2.5	11–11	6.5
8–0	2.8	12–2	6.8
8–3	3.0	12–5	7.0
8–7	3.3	12–8	7.3
8–9	3.5	12–11	7.5
9–1	3.8	13–2	7.8
9–3	4.0	13–5	8.0
9–7	4.3	13–8	8.3
9–10	4.5	13–10	8.5
10–2	4.8	14–1	8.8

Source: G. Thomas and I. Cresimbeni. *Guiding the Gifted Child* (New York: Random House, 1966), p. 36.

Extensive psychometric studies have established the average reading level expectancy for children of different ages. Thomas and Cresimbeni (1966) report grade equivalent expectancies derived from statistical norms on the Stanford Achievement Test, Iowa Every-Pupil Test, California Test of Mental Maturity—Primary Series, California Capacity Questionnaire, Gates Primary Reading Test, and Gates Reading Survey for grades 3 to 19. Similar reading level expectancies are derived by Jastak and Jastak (1976) from a population of more than fifteen thousand persons. An excerpt of the Thomas and Cresimbeni findings is presented in Table 5, which is a condensation of data for grades 1 through 8.

A close examination of Table 5 shows that the average child beginning first grade has a normal chronological and mental age of six years and two months. If a child eight years and seven months old and attending the third grade had a functional mental age of seven, we would not be surprised to find that he or she was achieving only on the high first-grade level. On the other hand, if we find that a boy whose mental and chronological age is nine years and seven months reads at the low second-grade level, we can assume that he has a significant reading disability. Both intelligence and mental age must be considered in determining reading expectancy.

Accordingly, several formulas for determining expected reading grade level are proposed by Bond and Tinker (1957), Dunn (1963), and Powell and Chansky (1967). Although these formulas vary somewhat, there is agreement that mental age and intelligence are the major factors; but that other factors, such as motivation, cultural background, self-concept, and practice, must be considered. For children who are experiencing great difficulty with the basic perceptual-linguistic skills usually acquired in kindergarten and the first and second grades, the following formula is helpful. RGE : M.A. minus 5 years, 3 months.

To interpret: reading grade expectancy (RGE) approximates mental age (M.A.) minus five years and three months. Since most children begin kindergarten at about five years old and progress through the grades chronologically, these expectations are reflected in Table 5. This formula is easy to apply but must be used with caution, as the margin of error in mental age scores and related statistical calculations must be taken into consideration. Jastak and Jastak (1976, pp. 44–45) report that when mental ability is held constant, girls significantly exceed boys (about .2 grade placement) in reading and spelling *at all grade levels*. This means that we should expect higher reading achievement scores from girls than from boys of the same ability.

Individual mental age scores are usually available to diagnostic-prescriptive specialists or can be derived from intelligence quotients using the formula [IQ = (M.A./C.A.) × 100] (Anastasi 1976, p. 84).

Example 1: Allen Williams
Chronological age of 8 years, 9 months
Mid-third-grade school placement
Mental age of 8 years, 7 months

$$IQ\ (98) = \frac{M.A.\ (103\ months)}{C.A.\ (105\ months)} \times 100$$

If chronological age and IQ are known, mental age can be determined using the formula [M.A. = C.A.x(IQ/100)].

Example 2: Susan Lamb
Chronological age of 7 years, 6 months
Low-second-grade school placement
Intelligence Quotient of 104

$$M.A.\ (7\ years,\ 10\ months) = C.A.\ (90\ months) \times \frac{IQ\ (104)}{100}$$

Naturally it is best to discover children with potential handicaps as soon as they enter school or at least in the first grade, since failure and frustration increase their inabilities and widen the gap between potential and performance. At the very least we must identify those who have fallen two years behind, since a greater setback may be irremediable.

DETERMINING SPECIFIC READING SKILL DEFICIENCIES

Specific skill deficiencies must be determined through both task and test analysis. The observant teacher can see problems in word-attack skills, contextual analysis, attention, comprehension, and other decoding skills by watching and listening to the child read and by maintaining a brief anecdotal record of functional errors and mistakes.

It is also possible for the teacher to conduct surveys of reading abilities, such as the following survey of phonetic and auditory readiness skills.

Consonant sounds

Look at these letters and tell me what sound you would make for them.

b l j c f p r n d m

Consonant blends

br sp th fl pr sh st dr pl

Syllables

ate er ing ed ow en ly

Synthesis

Name the second sound in the word **cat**.

Which sound in the word **stop** comes after **t**?

What word is made by putting these letters together: **m** then **a** then **n**?

Tell me the names and sounds of the letters in the word **dog.**

BASIC AUDITORY SKILLS SURVEY

Decoding   Listen carefully and then say the sounds I say.

                    T–T / pan–ban / b–k / cl–cl / lame–tame

               What letter do you hear at the beginning of these words?

                    girl   **f**ather   **t**oy   **p**lease   **k**iss   **s**tep

Rhyming   What rhymes with: boy   run   pop.

               Repeat after me

                    Mary had a little lamb,
                    Its fleece was white as snow,
                    And everywhere that Mary went
                    The lamb was sure to go.

               Watch me and slap your leg like I do.
               Good, now close your eyes and do it.

                    slap   slap / slap / slap   slap
                    slap   slap / slap slap slap / slap slap
                    (shave and a haircut two-bits pattern)

               I'm going to tap the desk with my knuckles like this (demonstrate). Close your eyes, listen carefully, and then tell me how many taps you hear. (The evaluator should make an irregular pattern of three, seven, and nine different taps.)

Memory   Repeat these sounds after me

                    5–7–9   1–a–buh   4–3–9–t
                    6–O–5–Y–7   2–Z–5–8–Q–3

BASIC VISUAL SKILLS SURVEY

Coordination

Look at the arrows below. Read the direction of the arrow and then move your eyes–not your head–in that direction.

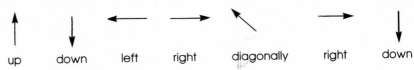

up   down   left   right   diagonally   right   down

Tracking

Look at, but do not touch, the numbers and letters on the line below and tell me what the first one is called (**M**). Good–now skip every other one and tell me the name of each symbol you see as fast as you can.

M 3 T   7 X   5 2 B C 1 A 4 D W Y 6 P Z

Integration

Look at, but do not touch, the symbols below. How many stars do you see (9)?

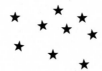

How many letter H's do you see (15)?

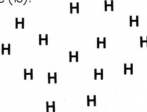

Look at the letters below. When you put them all together what does the word spell (father)?

F   A   T   H   E   R

Now look again and tell me two little words that you can find that are a part of that bigger word (fat, at, the, her).

Closure

Complete the following pictures in your mind and tell me what they are.

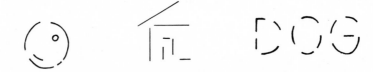

Kinesthetic-
Rhythmic
Integration

Watch how I tap out a pattern on the table with my knuckles–then you do it.

Patterns: . . / . . . / . . / . . .

. . / . / . . / . / . . / . . .

This time I want you to tap a simple pattern for me to copy. Watch carefully how we both do it because when I am done I want you to write down the pattern you made (using dot patterns as above).

Tactile
Discrimination

Close your eyes and concentrate on counting to yourself the number of times I tap on your back with my finger. (Make two, ten, and fourteen irregular taps and ask the child how many taps he or she felt each time.)

I am going to place your hand on top of mine. Now close your eyes and using your finger tap the back of my hand twelve times.

Visual-Motor
Integration and
Orientation

Take this piece of paper, put it on your forehead like this, then close your eyes and use this felt pen to print your first name on the paper.

Now take this sheet of paper on the desk, close your eyes, and print or write your first name for me.

In addition to task analysis and teacher surveys, reading tests, such as the Spache Diagnostic Reading Scales and the Stanford Diagnostic Reading Tests, have subtests that can be used for detailed analysis. The point is to determine major processing deficiencies since different remedial strategies are required for visual, auditory, or multisensory integration disabilities.

There are also several special criterion-referenced surveys available to help the diagnostician determine more specific processing deficiencies. We list these by skill areas:

Auditory Processing Skills.

Language-Structured Auditory Retention Span Test (Academic Therapy Publications) evaluates short-term auditory memory of unfamiliar words in sentences.

Wepman Auditory Discrimination Test (Joseph Wepman) is a brief test containing a list of forty similar and identical words for use in evaluating sound discrimination.

The Screening Test for Auditory Perception (Academic Therapy Publications) assesses vowel sounds, blends, rhythmic patterns, memory, and discrimination skills.

The Goldman-Fristoe-Woodcock Auditory Skills Test Battery (American Guidance Service) is a widely used comprehensive battery of tests for the assessment of auditory skills.

Visual Processing Skills.

The Hooper Visual Organization Test (Western Psychological Services) has thirty segmented pictures of common objects that require visual integration and organization by children of upper elementary age.

The 3-D Test for Visualization Skill (Academic Therapy Publications) uses solid geometric shapes to evaluate the child's spatial balance, memory, perception, and related skills.

Multisensory Skills.

The Jordan Left-Right Reversal Test (Academic Therapy Publications) measures the frequency of letter and number reversals.

Frostig Developmental Test of Visual Perception (Consulting Psychologists Press) is a visual-motor test that measures eye-hand coordination and perception of spatial relationship in paper and pencil tasks.

Illinois Test of Psycholinguistic Abilities (ITPA) (University of Illinois Press) includes twelve subtests: auditory reception, auditory association, auditory memory, auditory closure, visual association, visual closure, visual memory, visual reception, grammatical closure, sound blending, manual expression, and verbal expression. Although subtest scores are of questionable validity, this is a useful clinical test for special educators.

Slingerland Tests of Specific Language Disability (Educators Publishing Service) include nine different subtests that evaluate basic visual, auditory, and visual-motor skills using letters, words, numbers, sentences, and related symbols. Three different forms cover criterion tasks from grades 1 through 4.

The Psychoeducational Inventory of Basic Learning Abilities (Fearon Pitman Publishers) is a developmental series of motor, sensory, perceptual, language, and cognitive tasks. The tasks help in selecting and ranking objectives. A task analysis of student performance on the inventory and accompanying workbook must be supplemented with results from standardized tests.

Proper assessment of auditory, visual, linguistic, and related multisensory skill deficiencies requires a clinical task analysis of information derived from several sources. Jordan's *Dyslexia in the Classroom* (1972), with numerous case illustrations, is a good reference for the teacher interested in conducting specific task analysis of criterion tests for dyslexic children. Jordan shows how the results of auditory, visual, and related processing-skill tests can be directly used in the classroom or clinic.

DETERMINING NEUROPSYCHOLOGICAL DYSFUNCTION

The most significant indicators of neuropsychological dysfunction are to be found in test patterns showing poor sensory and psycholinguistic integration. Although difficulties in processing skills, such as visual-motor sequencing and organization, may lead to poor reading, writing, and related school performance, further assessment must be done outside the classroom to confirm these findings. Confirmation of findings requires individual neuropsychological assessment by a psychologist or physician who must then establish clinical evidence of the underlying factors in order to diagnose dyslexia.

Some of the instruments used by psychologists and diagnostic-prescriptive educators to detect neuropsychological dysfunction are listed below. All of the behavioral tasks required by these tests draw on the basic regulatory sensory-integrative functions that are necessary for higher psycholinguistic processing.

The Bender Gestalt Test for Children (Western Psychological Services) is a set of nine developmental figures for evaluating visual-motor organization and integration.

The Purdue Perceptual-Motor Survey (Charles E. Merrill Publishing Company) is a survey of balance, posture, body image and differentiation, perceptual-motor match, ocular control, and form perception.

The Harris Tests of Lateral Dominance (Psychological Corporation) include a series of eye, hand, and foot tasks to determine left/right-hemispheric dominance.

The Quick Neurological Screening Test (Academic Therapy Publications) assesses sensory loss, muscle coordination, and auditory and visual deficiencies.

Southern California Sensory Integration Tests (Western Psychological Services) are seventeen standardized tests measuring visual, tactile, kinesthetic, and motor performance.

The Bender-Purdue Reflex Test and Training Manual (Academic Therapy Publications) is for assessment of the labyrinthine, asymmetric, and symmetric tonic reflexes in young children.

Hyperactive Rating Scales (Fearon Pitman Publishers) are for use by parents and teachers in evaluating impulsiveness, poor attention span, excessive body movement, and related behaviors.

Clinical Evaluation of Sensory Integrative Dysfunction, in *Sensory Integration and Learning Disorders* (Ayres 1973), gives clinical procedures for evaluating primitive postural reflexes, muscle tone, vestibular system functioning, and body integration and control.

Luria's Neuropsychological Investigation (Christensen 1975) is a detailed manual for psychologists that includes assessment of auditory, visual, linguistic, and specific reading and writing skills.

Clinical neuropsychological investigation differs from traditional psychometric evaluation by purporting, as Christensen says,

> to analyze the defects qualitatively instead of quantitatively and is not based on preconceived classifications of functions derived from factor analysis but is instead directed towards investigations of the *organization* of mental processes (Christensen 1975, p. 23).

Geschwind (1962) explains how occlusion of the corpus callosum may lead to word blindness and how maldevelopment of the angular gyrus blocks the processing of visual language (which may result in dyslexia), but these defects must be inferred from the results of detailed clinical evaluation of auditory, visual, and sensory integrative behaviors.

Birch and Belmont (1965) establish that auditory-visual integration of rhythmic patterns (such as tapping on a table top) is related to reading performance in the primary grades. This study helps to establish the importance of rhythmic patterning as a neuropsychological behavior to be evaluated in the diagnosis of dyslexia. A study by Satz and Friel (1974) of 497 kindergarten children demonstrates the predictive ability of neuropsychological tests of sensory-perceptual-motor skills (such as finger localization, visual-auditory discrimination, and verbal recitation tasks) on actual reading achievement. Mutti, Sterling, Spalding, and Crawford (1974) studied 176 children and found a highly significant statistical disparity between ordinary and learning-disabled children on neurological impairment scores derived from ten clinical sensory-motor and perceptual tests.

Recent studies by Ayres (1978) measure the duration of nystagmus following rotation among learning-disabled children. Those children with vestibular disorders show hyperactive postrotary nystagmus. For example, when children are spun around ten to fifteen times with their eyes closed and then abruptly stopped, their eyes normally display a rapid horizontal reflexive movement. Prolonged (hyperreactive) nystagmus may reflect less than normal inhibition from higher levels of the brain upon the vestibular nuclei in the brain stem. With sensory integrative (vestibular, tactile, and proprioceptive) stimulation and training, academic performance improves and the duration of nystagmus is reduced.

Below are some specific tasks used by psychologists and physicians to evaluate neuropsychological integration and organization.

Eye Tracking.   Hold your head still and follow the eraser on this pencil. (The pencil is held about eighteen inches from the eyes.)

Thumb and Finger Circles.   Make a circle with your thumb and finger like this. Now touch each finger to your thumb. Now do it with your other hand.

Finger to Nose.   Touch the tip of your nose like this. Now touch my hand and close your eyes and touch your nose. Now do it with the other hand.

Rapid Hand Movements.   Put your hands on your knees like this. Now turn them over with your palms up like this. Now continue to do it as fast as you can.

Simultaneous Touch.   Close your eyes and then touch the two places on your body that I touch.

Tandem Walk.   Put your heel against your toe and walk on this straight line. Now walk backwards in the same way. Now do it again with your eyes shut.

Arm and Leg Extension/Choreiform Movements.   Sit on this chair like this and put your arms and legs out, spread out your fingers, stick out your tongue, and hold it that way for a minute.

Standing Balance and Hop.   Stand on your right foot. Now your left foot. Now do it again with your eyes closed. Now hop twice on each foot.

Sterognosis.   Tell me what I place in your hand behind your back (coin, rubber band, tack, key).

Graphesthenia.   Close your eyes and tell me what letters I am drawing on your index finger (*o   a   c   s   v*).

Laterality.

Eye Preference
   paper telescope sighting
   hole-in-card sighting
   "rifle shooting" sighting

Foot Preference
    kicking a ball
    stepping on chair
    writing initials with foot
Hand Preference
    writing name
    throwing a paper ball
    using scissors
    simulating brushing teeth
    drawing developmental figures below

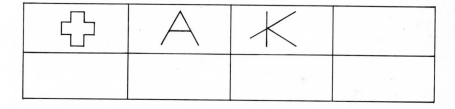

Ear Preference
    Cover your left ear with your left hand and listen carefully to what I whisper into your right ear. Then tell me what you hear.

	Left Ear	Right Ear
Digits:	1-6-3	3-1-6
	8-2-4-9	9-4-8-2
	2-9-5-O-7	7-O-5-2-9
	O-2-3-6-1-5	5-1-6-3-O-2
Blends:	fl-pr-sp	sp-fl-pr
	pl-st-br	br-st-pl
	sh-fl-sp-th	sh-fl-sp-th
	pl-fl-sp-dr	dr-pl-fl-sp
Syllables:	ing-er-ate	er-ate-ing
	ly-ic-ed	ic-ed-ly
	ow-it-en	en-it-ow

DETERMINING ASSOCIATED FACTORS

The major associated factors that produce primary reading disorders must also be investigated. One of these is the lack of student motivation and interest in reading. A teacher or parent should note any special reading interests such as magazines, hobby kits, or comics. Rewards for reading can help. Has the student received good marks, grades, praise, or recognition for reading? Many dyslexic boys actually work harder at reading than classmates, but they are seldom praised sufficiently for their efforts, and many of them give up and become convinced that they cannot read.

With other children gross sensory impairment (such as partial loss of sight or deafness) or ill health may cause reading disorders. A history of early childhood disease or such things as dizziness, car sickness, poor coordination in hitting and catching a ball or in other sports, ear infections, and other similar problems must be considered. Such health difficulties as chronic malnourishment may seriously affect a child's performance.

Fear and anxiety usually accompany history of failure at reading tasks. Anxiety and related emotional disorders usually diminish and disappear with prescriptive-remedial instruction and accomplishment. Sometimes however, personal and family problems may be responsible for acute anxiety and distraction and may require social work or psychological investigation and intervention.

SUMMARY

The diagnostic summary on page 84 includes the seven areas that must be examined when attempting to diagnose a child who is suspected of being dyslexic.

The Individual Profile of Learning Skills and Abilities shown on page 86 has been found useful as a means of summarizing available test results. The student's age and grade expectancy should be circled and all scores written on the profile form. When completed, the profile will show relative strengths and weaknesses in each developmental area and can be used in diagnostic-prescriptive planning.

DISCUSSION QUESTIONS AND ACTIVITIES

1. Conduct a functional reading assessment of a child using basal readers as suggested by Spache. Present and discuss your findings.

2. List some other skills that might be added to those in Table 4.

3. Visit an elementary school and study the current group reading tests being used. Write a report on when and how they are used.

4. Using the multiple-choice format of the Stanford Diagnostic Reading Test, write a thirty-minute lesson based on one of the seven subtests.

5. Use available group reading test results to make a diagnostic profile on a reading-disabled child.

6. Select and discuss an individual diagnostic reading test not mentioned in this chapter.

7. Administer the Peabody Picture Vocabulary Test to a reading-disabled child and interpret its results relative to the WISC subtest scores provided you by the school psychologist.

8. Give the reading grade expectancy (RGE) for the following children and explain how you arrived at your answers:
   Boy: M.A.   7 years, 9 months
   Girl: M.A. 10 years, 3 months
   Boy: M.A.   5 years, 5 months
   Girl: M.A.   7 years, 9 months

9. Calculate mental age scores for the following children:
   Billy Smith: C.A. 8 years; IQ 92
   Gail Brown: C.A. 7 years, 11 months; IQ 108

10. What is the RGE for Billy Smith and Gail Brown?

11. At what functional reading level would Billy and Gail be determined to have a significant reading disability?

12. Explain how you might arrive at the conclusion that Billy or Gail could have a significant reading disability.

13. Supplement the Phonetic Readiness Survey (p. 72) and the Basic Auditory Skills Survey (p. 73) with other tasks. Administer them to a reading-disabled child and interpret your findings.

14. Determine the specific reading skill deficiencies of a reading-disabled student using several of the individual processing skill tests described in this chapter.

15. Cooperate with the psychologist in the diagnostic evaluation of a child suspected of being dyslexic. What neuropsychological tests and tasks were used to determine dyslexic dysfunction and what were the results?

16. Describe how a child's improper school placement and inappropriate education might produce an acute anxiety reaction and exacerbate a dyslexic syndrome.

DYSLEXIA DIAGNOSTIC SUMMARY

Student's Name _____   Birthdate _____   C.A. _____

Teacher _____   Current Grade-level Placement _____

1. Functional Reading Level

	Tests Used	Grade Placement	Standard Score
Classroom basal reading group			
Oral paragraph comprehension			
Silent paragraph comprehension			
Oral vocabulary			
Phonic skills			
Estimated total functional reading performance			

2. Reading Potential

Listening-to-story grade-level comprehension_____

WISC Full Scale IQ _____   Verbal Scale _____   Performance Scale _____

Mental age _____   Mental age reading expectancy _____

3. Significant Reading Disability

Mental age reading grade-level expectancy   _____

Total functional reading grade level   _____

Discrepancy   _____

Does a significant discrepancy of approximately two or more years exist? ____

Comments _____

continued

4. **Specific Processing Skill Deficiencies**

Auditory_____   Mechanics _____   Cognitive-programming dysfunctions _____

Visual _____

- ☐ Omissions
- ☐ Reversals

- ☐ Comprehension
- ☐ Contextual

Multisensory _____

- ☐ Repetitions
- ☐ Additions
- ☐ Word attack
- ☐ Guesses

Comments _____

5. **Neuropsychological Dysfunctions**   Regulation   Processing   Programming

6. **Associated Factors**   Motivation   Anxiety   Health   Reinforcement

7. **Developmental-Remedial Strategies**   Priority objectives   Learning tasks

INDIVIDUAL PROFILE OF LEARNING SKILLS AND ABILITIES

Name		Grade		CA		MA

APPROXIMATE GRADE EXPECTANCY

GRADE:	LK	MK	HK	L1	H1	L2	H2	L3	M3	L4	M4	L5	M5	H5	M6	L7	M7	L8	M8	L9	M9	L10
AGE:	5	5½	6	6½	7	7½	8	8½	9	9½	10	10½	11	11½	12	12½	13	13½	14	14½	15	15½

	Skills and Abilities	Comments/Other Criterion Evaluations	Profile (percentile/standard)				
			Very Low	Below Average	Average	Above Average	Very High
Gross Motor Abilities	Balance						
	Coordination						
	Strength						
	Other						
Sensory-motor Abilities	Attention-concentration (WISC-DS)						
	Laterality						
	Manual expression (ITPA)						
	Other						
Auditory Perception	Auditory reception (ITPA)						
	Auditory association (ITPA)						
	Auditory sequential memory (ITPA)						
	Auditory closure (ITPA)						
	Sound blending (ITPA)						
	Consonant sounds (Spache)						
	Vowel sounds (Spache)						
	Consonant blends (Spache)						
	Common syllables (Spache)						
	Other						
Visual Perception	Visual form constancy (Frostig)						
	Visual position in space (Frostig)						
	Visual figure ground (Frostig)						
	Visual closure (ITPA)						
	Visual reception (ITPA)						
	Visual memory (WISC-PC)						
	Visual association (ITPA)						
	Other						
Visual-motor Perception	Eye-hand coordination (Frostig)						
	Spatial relations (Frostig)						
	Visual sequential memory (ITPA)						

	Skills and Abilities	Comments/Other Criterion Evaluations	Profile (percentile/standard)				
			Very Low	Below Average	Average	Above Average	Very High
Visual-motor Perception (continued)	Visual motor planning (WISC mazes)						
	Visual motor synthesis (WISC BD)						
	Object assembly (WISC)						
	Fine motor control (WISC code)						
	Visual motor integration Bender VM Gestalt						
	Other						
Language Abilities	Verbal expression (ITPA)						
	Receptive vocabulary (PPVT)						
	Expressive vocabulary (WISC/Binet)						
	Grammatic closure (ITPA)						
	Oral reading vocabulary (WRAT/Spache)						
	Oral reading comprehension (Spache)						
	Silent reading comprehension (Spache)						
	Spelling (WRAT)						
	Other						
Conceptual-cognitive Abilities	General information (WISC)						
	Comprehension and reasoning (WISC)						
	Similarities and abstractions (WISC)						
	Functional mental age (WISC/Binet)						
	Arithmetic reasoning (WISC)						
	Arithmetic operations (WRAT)						
	Other						
Social-personal Abilities	Self identification (DAP)						
	Social planning and anticipation (WISC PA)						
	Social maturity (Vineland SA)						
	Self esteem						
	Behavior ratings						
	Other						

Special Education

Change in practice as a result of
research occurs only if teachers in
some way become aware of the
findings of pertinent investigations.
Ira Aaron

CHAPTER SIX

Experiments in Sensory-Motor Education and Reading

In this and the following chapters we will be mainly concerned with selective research that focuses on severely reading-disabled children who appear to have primary neuropsychological processing dysfunctions. Our major concern is to consider gains made as a result of *neuropsychological education*. For our purposes, neuropsychological education is construed as a form of training that tries to change or improve brain functioning and operation through special exercises, tasks, and prescriptive learning activities.

Four major categories of neuropsychological education will be considered eventually, but this chapter deals with sensory-motor organization and integration.

APPLIED CLINICAL THEORY

In educational practice, Maria Montessori (1964) was one of the first workers to hypothesize that the mind can be made to grow and develop through the use of special educational methods, such as manipulative cognitive games and related sensory-motor games, but it was not for many years that special education was aimed more directly at neurological intervention and remediation. More recently special educators began to adapt the extensive clinical studies in physical therapy and rehabilitation to the needs of the special school and classroom.

Semans (1959) summarizes research showing how various sensory stimulation techniques affect the reticular facilitory and inhibitory systems. Some of the educational methods and tasks used in these investigations include volitional and nonvolitional (directed) placement of the arms and legs, body righting–equilibrium activities, and the patterning of movements.

The fundamental premise in sensory-motor education and treatment is that a human nervous system that is impeded in its development may and must be given opportunities to strengthen its functions if serious developmental and reading problems are to be prevented. The marriage of theory and practice is illustrated by this statement:

> Cortical hemispheric dominance is a result of function. Consistent use of a single hand develops the controlling hemisphere and will result in speech. Continued use of a single hand at near point, such as with drawing, will also help establish eyedness; this results in writing (Delacato 1966, p. 41).

BODY ORGANIZATION

Body organization theory, research, and practice follow the premise that superimposed and structured sensory and motor activities help to make the body better organized and have a direct influence on neurological organization centers of the brain itself. Many different kinds of body organization programs and experiments have been conducted and few of them establish the value of *isolated* training in improving reading performance. Some studies, however, include sensory-motor training along with other kinds of education and are worthy of consideration.

Delacato (1966) conducted an experimental study in which forty-three kindergarten children in a sensory-motor neurological organization program were contrasted with forty-one control group children. The experimental program consisted of seven daily sessions (five to fifteen minutes each) of creeping and cross-pattern walking activities plus two daily sessions (twenty-five minutes each) of listening to nursery rhymes, stories, and folk songs. The experimental group demonstrated over twice the gain of controls in visual discrimination, attention span, and reading-readiness scores.

The neurologist LeWinn (1969) summarizes a number of studies showing that neurological maturation and organization require environmental challenge, stimulation, demands, and specific opportunity for functional development of dendritic processes, glial multiplication, and the growth of cortical tissue. In an earlier study, Doman (1960) and his colleagues attempted to improve neurological organization in children with severe brain injuries through the use of gross-motor and sensory stimulation tasks. Seventy-six children with a median age of thirty months were involved in a two-year experiment of crawling and patterning. The "patterning" attempted to impose patterns of body movement on the children. Further sensory-motor stimulation consisted of brushing, pinching, and so forth. Although this was a clinical study, highly significant gains in mobility were reported for some children, and researchers suspected that language gains were made. This study is controversial and has not been substantiated in other research. Even so, many of the sensory-motor techniques in this and related studies have long been used in special education and remain of value if appropriately used.

The most appropriate use of gross-sensory training activities is to relate them directly to symbolic learning. This link can be made through motor and sensory games and lessons. Many of these have been in use since Montessori's time but have been modified. A group of sensory-motor lessons and exercises appears at the end of this chapter.

SENSORY DISCRIMINATION

Most sensory-motor training programs provide many multisensory discrimination activities. In these lessons, body movement and organization are combined with other tactual, kinesthetic, and perceptual skills, although the emphasis is on gross discrimination tasks.

A study reported by Miracle (1966) assesses the linguistic effects of neuropsychological techniques in the treatment of a selected group of retarded readers. The group consisted of forty fourth- and fifth-grade students at least one year behind in both vocabulary and reading on the Iowa Test of Basic Skills. The experimental program consisted of remedial reading with sensory-motor activities and produced significant improvement in reading scores over the control group. The controls received no remediation and adjustment was made for the Hawthorne effect (significant results caused by new or different procedure). Of equal importance was the finding that the experimental group demonstrated more interest in reading than the controls.

Mariam (1966) found that successful programs of this type used the following remedial methods:

- word-attack drills with phonic instruction
- free library reading
- reading accelerators and controlled readers
- eye-hand coordination, tracking, fixation tasks
- cross-pattern walking and crawling games
- stereo reader material to strengthen the preferred eye

Painter (1966) conducted a similar experiment with kindergarten children in which twenty-one half-hour training sessions were held over a seven-week period. These sessions emphasized rhythmic activities (drum tapping, moving to the sound of a metronome, generalization of rhythmic patterns), visual and auditory discrimination, kinesthetic-tactual awareness, and flexibility. The children made significant gains on the ITPA motor encoding and the auditory-vocal association subtest.

Faustman (1968) reports on the effects of an integrated Frostig/ Strauss/Kephart/Winterhaven sensory-motor and perceptual training program conducted with kindergarten children. The one-year experiment involved fourteen experimental and fourteen control classes (all of normal intelligence). In addition to such activities as rhythms, design matching, visual discrimination, and object manipulation and classification, language experience units were developed around the material used. In first grade the experimental group was superior in both perceptual scores and word recognition achievement on the Gates Primary Word Recognition Test.

Heber (1972) and his colleagues report on an eight-year longitudinal follow-up of twenty "high risk retarded children" who were provided with intensive sensory-motor, language, and problem-solving activities. Results showed the experimental group to be reading significantly earlier and better than either retarded controls or nonretarded children of the same grade level, and this advantage continued through the fourth grade.

VESTIBULAR ORIENTATION

A few sensory-motor training programs include activities to develop vestibular-righting reflexes with the assumption that this will improve total neurological integration. In one such study, Ayres (1972) conducted a sensory-integration experiment with 148 children with postural, ocular, and bilateral integration problems; apraxis; form-space difficulties; auditory-language disorders; and laterality disturbances. Finally selecting thirty experimental and thirty control-group children, Ayres instituted a unique sensory-motor program. Training activities included visual-spatial games, sensory-integration vestibular orienting activities (such as scooters, swings, bouncing boards), and rhythm and music. She theorized that, among other things, extra ocular muscular control would develop, resulting in increased efficiency of the attentional mechanisms of the right hemisphere and better communication with the left hemisphere's language center. Her experimental group made significant gains on the Wide Range Achievement Test Reading scores. Ayres (1973) has also developed an extensive manual of sensory-motor integration therapy, which emphasizes tactile and vestibular stimulation and presents numerous multilearning activities for use with young children.

Much applied sensory-motor research has been done by Cratty at the University of California, Los Angeles. Working with a great variety of reading- and learning-disabled children, Cratty (1970) compiled and evaluated research studies showing the importance of movement and sensory education for improving attention and academic learning. Much of this research has been compiled for use by teachers, including lessons combining active learning and stimulation with specific reading and intellectual skills (Cratty 1971, 1973).

BEVERLY–A BRAIN-DAMAGED CHILD

Beverly was a girl of eight and a half who was a good student in a public school. She was involved in an automobile accident that resulted in significant brain damage and extensive hospitalization.

Beverly was comatose for some time. When she regained consciousness she showed a loss of both speech (aphasia) and reading (alexia). When her special education began, assessment disclosed spatial orientation difficulties, confusion of body parts and laterality, poor balance and directionality, no sense of time orientation, poor rhythm, and complete loss of visual-auditory decoding skills. These were all diagnosed as critical sensory-motor integration skills, the development of which were prerequisites for higher-order perceptual and linguistic functioning. Following remedial and developmental procedures described by Valett (1974), Beverly received more than sixty individual prescriptive teaching sessions and twenty-two group activity sessions of approximately forty-five minutes each. She was then returned to the formal school program.

Beverly's early sensory-motor training focused on target crawling, jumping and rhythm games, symbol-throwing activities, spatial orientation and organization of concrete objects including wooden symbols, and a series of auditory-phonics tasks. Gradually her sensory-motor integration began to improve and the emphasis in training was switched to more advanced perceptual-linguistic tasks. Eventually Beverly relearned to read and perform academically, although not on a normal expectancy level.

Similarly, Luria's extensive work with brain-damaged patients demonstrates in great detail how brain functions can be restored following injury with the use of exercises, occupational therapy, and special reeducation techniques. Luria found that restoration of brain function involved the radical reorganization of the destroyed or impaired activity by means of transfer and development of different but associated neuronal structures. Movement and rhythmic tasks were determined to be critical for relearning spatial orientation and psycholinguistic operations (Luria 1963).

Other clinical and experimental research with both children and adults confirms the value of highly prescriptive sensory-motor training in neuropsychological disorders. By itself, however, such training is of limited value and must be combined with higher-order neuropsychological education if it is to be effective in the remediation of severe reading disorders.

INSTRUCTIONAL MATERIALS

It is apparent from developmental remedial programs, such as those by Faustman, Heber, Ayres, and others, that sensory-motor training is most effective when it requires the integration and organization of varied sensory input and results in some form of symbolic or linguistic output. Fine auditory and visual discrimination, good rhythm and motor coordination, sequential memory, speed, and efficiency are required in many higher-order linguistic tasks such as writing.

Many new educational toys and games are manufactured that are of value in developing the sensory-motor readiness skills required in more advanced academic learning. Companies such as Child Guidance Toys produce numerous sensory-motor materials that have been used successfully in early childhood and special education programs. These materials can be obtained in toy or department stores or through school supply houses.

More recently, a number of new electronic games and instructional materials have been produced that appear quite promising for use in sensory-motor education. Most of these materials emit a combination of visual, auditory, kinesthetic, and symbolic cues that must be integrated to solve selected problems. Three widely used examples follow:

Simon (Milton Bradley Company).   This game uses a large, dish-shaped piece of plastic with four colored panels (red, green, blue, yellow). When the starting button is pressed, one of the colored panels lights up and a tone is emitted. Then, if the player responds by pressing that panel correctly, *Simon* adds another colored panel light and tone. The object is to remember the sequence of lights and tones and to press as many panels as possible. If a player mistakes the sequence, *Simon* produces a "razz" sound. Different levels of difficulty can be selected ranging from one to thirty-one memory sequences. Players may play against *Simon,* themselves, or others. The four colored panels can also be numbered and labeled with number or alphabet sequences. Students can then write down the sequences on paper (such as 1, 3, 2, 4—A, D, C, B—red, red, blue, green, yellow, yellow). This activity is another form of rehearsal and feedback for improving sequential memory.

Comp IV (Milton Bradley Company).   This is a challenging computer numbers game. It uses a small console with nine numbers and a readout display window. The object of the game is to determine a number sequence preselected by the computer. The sequences range in difficulty from two to nine digits as selected by the player. Numbers are punched into the computer and the display window gives visual feedback as to the correctness of the numbers and their sequence.

Merlin (Parker Brothers).   This is a most versatile instrument in that six different games may be played that demand varying levels of audio, visual, and kinesthetic integration. The instrument is similar in size to a portable tape recorder and has nine numbered input buttons and a selector panel. The games include single Tic-Tac-Toe, Music Machine (reading and playing computer music), Echo (repeating lights and tones in correct sequence), and other more difficult games requiring logical analysis and synthesis.

Each of the above electronic games is relatively inexpensive and available in almost all communities. Other similar games are available on special interest areas such as football, but require some reading and knowledge of rules of the game. It can be expected that many other instructional materials of value to special educators will be developed in the near future.

SUMMARY

In this chapter we have discussed the use of sensory-motor training in the remediation of severe reading and language problems. Sensory-motor training is a kind of neuropsychological education that focuses on the development of regulatory brain-unit functional skills, such as attention, inhibition, and gross sensory discrimination and organization.

Critical sensory-motor abilities include body organization, spatial orientation, rhythm and balance, time and speed regulation, lateral consistency, and tactual-kinesthetic discrimination. All of these skills and abilities can be developed and related to the reading process.

For the neuropsychologically impaired child sensory-motor education is essential and may be intensive and prolonged. To be most effective for the dyslexic child, such training must provide direct practice with the sensory-motor integration and discrimination of psycholinguistic symbols. Since this kind of prescriptive education is not essential for children who are progressing normally in academic learning, it should be used with discrimination by classroom teachers.

SENSORY-MOTOR LESSONS

Following are eleven exercises that combine a single sensory-motor activity with some form of symbolic learning. These exercises might prove helpful in the reeducation of brain-damaged children, or as a first step in the education of children with impaired brain function.

Objective: to coordinate one's crawling and body movements in pursuit of a target

Materials: pencil, ball, book, chalk path, symbol cards

Directions: Look at the drawing of a child crawling toward the book. Now look at the chalk line on the floor. You are to start crawling on the X mark and move quickly to the book. If necessary I will help you. Stay on the chalk mark. We will also time how long it takes you to reach the book.

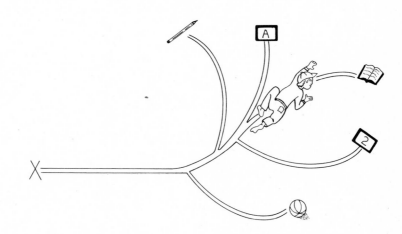

Evaluation:

Tries	Time
1	
2	
3	

Variations: Add more objects, make a more difficult path, have the child make the path and choose the objects. Crawl to sequences of symbol cards.

Objective: to be able to place one's body in specified positions and to coordinate movements

Materials: picture cards, chalk

Directions: Look at this picture card of a swimmer:

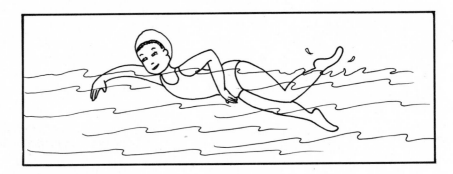

- Show me how a swimmer moves his head, arms, and hands. I will help you if necessary.
- Pretend that you are swimming. Swim over to that wall and back and show me how you move your arms and hands.
- Now pretend you are swimming backstroke and make your arms and head move together like this (demonstrate).
- Pretend you are swimming in a large figure 8 like this chalk design on the floor. Now you do it and change your strokes as you move around the figure 8.
- Swim the figure 8 again but this time call out "left" or "right" as you move each arm.

Evaluation:

Tries	+	+ /−	−	Time
1				
2				
3				

Variations: Go to a swimming pool and actually teach the varied strokes and techniques. Have the child act and move like a bear, snake, or elephant. Make letters **C, F, I, P, Y,** and so forth.

Objective: to select and crawl a symbol sequence

Materials: three symbol cards and chalk designs

Directions: Look at these three symbol cards:

This one is called a circle:

This one is called a triangle:

This one is called the letter **B**:

Now you tell me their names.

Look at the floor where each symbol has been drawn in chalk. You are to crawl over each symbol as quickly as you can beginning with the circle, then moving to the triangle and finally the letter **B**. Tell me the order in which you are going to go.

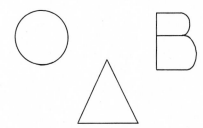

Evaluation:

Tries	Time
1	
2	
3	

Variations: Have the child select the order of symbols, add other symbols, overlap the symbols.

Objective: to move rhythmically to a nursery rhyme

Materials: a picture book of nursery rhymes

Directions: Look at this book of rhymes. It reads:

Jack be nimble
Jack be quick
Jack jump over the candlestick.

Walk with me in a circle as we say the rhyme and feel the rhythm.

Good. Now this time when we get to the word **jump** we will jump and continue walking like this.

Now this time you say the rhyme, walk, and jump by yourself.

Evaluation:

Tries	+	Rhythm + / –	–
1			
2			
3			

Variations: Use other nursery rhymes. Have children select their own rhymes and vary the rhythms.

Objective: to balance and move one's body rhythmically while thinking aloud

Materials: trampoline, flash cards

Directions: Get up on the trampoline and bounce for awhile to get your balance.

Now bounce three times on your feet, then once on your seat, then three times on your feet, and so on. This time as you bounce, call out "feet, feet, feet, seat," "feet, feet, feet, seat."

Look at these cards. This time as you bounce I will show you a card and I want you to call out the letters or numbers that you see. Call out one for each bounce. Cards:

1	2	3	4	5	6	7

a	b	c	d	e	f	g

1	3	5	7	9	11

a	c	e	g	i	k	m

Evaluation:

Circle symbols correct

1	2	3	4	5	6	7
a	b	c	d	e	f	g
1	3	5	7	9	11	
a	c	e	g	i	k	m

Variations: Use cards with both letters and numbers, use words, and vary rhythm using a metronome.

Objective: to use the dominant foot in tracing and drawing symbols

Materials sand lot or dirt yard, design-symbol cards

Directions: Look at the designs on these cards. Take the first card and use your foot (dominant foot) to copy the design here in the dirt. Now do the other symbols one at a time.

Cards:

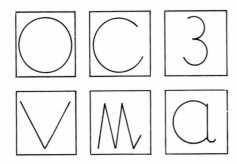

Evaluation:

Symbol	+	+ /-	-
O			
C			
3			
V			
M			
a			

Variations: Have the child pick a two- or three-card sequence and then make the designs from memory. Ask the child to create his or her own designs.

Objective:　　to trace symbols and words correctly and improve writing skills using the Perceptualmotor Pen

Materials:　　symbol cards, word cards, number cards, and the Perceptualmotor "Talking" Pen

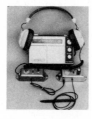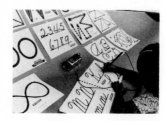

Directions:

1. Look at this device. It is called the "talking pen" because it operates on flashlight batteries and "talks" by making sounds when it is misused.

2. Here is a black circle. Turn the pen on like this and trace the circle. When you trace correctly the pen is quiet. Notice that when you move off the circle the pen makes a noise that warns you to get back on the lines.

3. Now we will put carbon paper between this sheet and some drawing paper. This time, as you trace the designs (below) listen carefully to the talking pen and try hard to stay on the lines. If you trace correctly, the design will show on the carbon copy, which we will check when you have finished.

4. Good. This time we will trace letters. Listen carefully to the talking pen and stay on the lines. Every time the pen makes a noise we will count one mistake and note it below each letter.

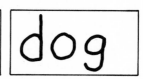

___　　___　　___　　___　___

continued

5. Trace the numbers below using the talking pen and then note the number of mistakes you have made.

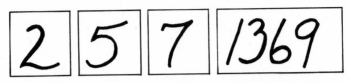

6. Now put this earphone on your **left** ear (the right hemisphere processes music). I am plugging the talking pen into this music converter. Retrace each of the symbols (in steps 3, 4 and 5 above) and notice that this time you will hear nice music as you stay on the lines. The music stops when you go off the lines. Look at your carbon copy and count the number of errors.

7. Now put the earphone on your right ear (for left hemisphere linguistic processing). We will put a clean sheet under the carbon paper. Turn up the volume and listen to the tape. This time retrace the designs with the talking pen and notice that when you get off the design a voice tells you to get back on. Look at your carbon copy and count your errors.

8. Continue to listen to this tape with your right earphone. I have dictated the designs that I want you to trace. Listen carefully and trace **only** those designs that you hear. When you go off the lines the pen will make a disagreeable sound. Try to trace them as accurately and as fast as you can.

Evaluation:

Task no.	Total number of errors		
	1st try	2nd try	3rd try
3			
4			
5			
6			
7			
8			

Variations:

Have the child trace names and addresses and reduce number of errors with practice. Use phrase cards from reading books or stories from the child's experience for copying. Use the talking pen to trace sentences or words dictated by the child and written in model form by the teacher.

Objective: to use vestibular orienting and righting reflexes in thinking and moving

Materials: a single rope tire swing

Directions: Look at the picture of this girl standing in the tire swing:

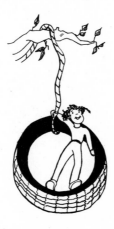

Now stand in the tire swing and get it to move back and forth.
See if you can move it in a straight line.
Now try to move it in a big circle.
Now make the circle go the other way.
Try to make it go in a big figure 8.
Now twist and spin the swing and count out loud to ten.

Evaluation:

Symbol	+	+ /-	-
↔			
↺			
↻			
∞			
Spin			

Variations: Move toward symbol targets placed in a circle around the swing; use rhymes and songs while moving.

SENSORY-MOTOR LESSON

Objective: to detect and verbalize symbols made on the back, arms, hands, and fingers

Materials: a camel's hair brush, electric vibrator, pencil, blindfold

Directions: I am going to blindfold you and then use this little brush to paint on the palm of your hand. Tell me what design or symbol I am making:

X   O   V

This time I will use the pencil to draw on the tip of your index finger. Tell me what design you think I am drawing:

O   C   I   H

Now I will use this vibrator and make large symbols on your back. Tell me what symbols I am making:

△   2   B   7

Evaluation:

Task	+	+ /-	-
hand			
finger			
back			

Variations: Pinch large symbols on the back or use an old toothbrush to change sensitivity; ask the child to draw what he or she feels.

Objective: to develop balance by skating

Materials: skate boards, beginning roller skates, regular roller skates

Directions: 1. **Skateboard**—Carefully place one foot on the skateboard like this and push away with your other foot. Stand on the board, skate across the room, and pick up the colored cloth target. Then turn around, skate back, and place the cloth on this chair.

2. **Beginning roller skates**—First, I want you just to stand and balance on both skates as I slowly push you around the room. Skate around by yourself and try to improve your balance. Now skate in a big circle around the whole room. I will time you to see how long it takes.

3. **Regular roller skates**—Now that you are using regular skates try these activities:

- skate to music
- skate with a partner to music
- figure skate making circles and figure 8s.

Evaluation:

Task	+	+ /–	–	Time
1				
2				
3				
Other				

Variations: Develop routines with special music, such as skating relay games, "Simon says," skating out number and letter forms, and ice skating.

Objective: to correctly integrate and reproduce a visual-auditory-kinesthetic sequence

Materials: **Simon** electronic game (Milton Bradley Company), paper, and pencil

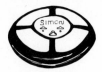

Directions: This is an electronic game called **Simon**. Put your finger on the yellow, green, red, and blue panels and name the colors as you touch them.

1. **Color-tone discrimination**–This first game is called **Simon says**. We switch **Simon** on, press the start button, and then watch a colored light panel light up and listen to the sound each light makes. Now you press the panels in the order that **Simon** lighted them. If you make a mistake **Simon** will give you a razz sound, and you can try again. If you get the entire sequence right **Simon** will reward you with a special sound and flashing lights. After you complete the sequence push the "last sequence" button and check your response.

2. **Color-naming**–This time we will play it again except that I want you to name the colors quietly to yourself as **Simon** lights them up and as you press out the sequence. When you finish the sequence write the first initial of each color in your sequence on the line below:

   _____

   Now push the "last sequence" button and check your responses written on the line above.

3. **Left-right integration**–We will play the same game except that this time your left hand will push the yellow and green panels and your right hand will push the red and blue panels. When you have finished write down the color sequence on the line below:

   _____

   Now push the "last sequence" button and check your response.

4. **Number sequence**–Look at each panel and notice that a number from one through four has been taped on each panel. Touch them and tell me each number. Again, use your left and right hands for this game. As **Simon** plays and you respond, say each number to yourself. When you have finished pressing out your sequence, write down the numbers on the line below and then push the "last sequence" button to check your response:

   _____

continued

5. **Letter sequence**–Notice that each of the panels also has a letter taped to it. Touch the **A,B,C,** and **D** and say their names to yourself. This time use both hands again and say the letters quietly to yourself as you watch **Simon** and as you repeat the letter sequence. When you have finished write down the letter sequence on the line below and then press the "last sequence" button to check your response:

_____

6. **Auditory-kinesthetic sequence**–Again, use your left hand for the yellow and green panels and your right hand for the red and blue panels. By this time you will have learned that a special tone sounds for each panel. **Close your eyes** and just listen to the tone sequence that **Simon** makes. Then open your eyes, look at the panels, and press out the correct tone sequence. When you have finished write your sequence below using the initials for each color and then press the "last sequence" button to check your response:

_____

Evaluation: Record each response as indicated above and carefully note the length of each sequence.

Variations: Have the student maintain a personal record of all written sequences. Provide extended practice in each sequence and reward extended memory sequences. Go on to more advanced sequences and games provided in the instructions to **Simon.**

DISCUSSION QUESTIONS AND ACTIVITIES

1. Define *neuropsychological education.*

2. Describe several different kinds of neuropsychological education and present some examples of each.

3. Look up and demonstrate some of the sensory-motor lessons developed by Montessori for use in language learning.

4. What is patterning? Discuss its proper use in special education and remedial therapy.

5. Demonstrate some specific sensory-motor skills and explain their relevance to the reading process.

6. Why might sensory-motor training be of particular value for young boys who are academically retarded?

7. Discuss the contributions of sensory-motor experiments in the development of attention, concentration, and interest in learning.

8. Research and discuss in detail the study by Heber. Include a review of currently available reports.

9. Discuss Ayres's study of sensory-motor integration training and its effect on reading test scores.

CHAPTER SEVEN

Remediating Visual Processing Deficiencies

Most neuropsychological education programs attempt to develop visual, auditory, and related multisensory abilities. Direct attempts are also made to *remediate* whatever specific processing dysfunctions may have been diagnosed. In this chapter we will concentrate on the visual processing skills of symbol discrimination, symbol tracking, visual organization, and visual memory.

Chalfant and Scheffelin (1969) discuss the importance of visual symbol processing as a key perceptual-linguistic function in reading. During the early years of childhood, visual association and language experience in meaningful social contacts are critical prerequisites for later, more symbolic forms of visual discrimination and interpretation. Gradually the visual process is refined, and, with appropriate practice, culturally correct responses to visual perception become habitual. Through experience we learn to improve our visual discriminations, to locate and track what we see and wish to follow, to organize our visual perceptions, and to recall and integrate our visual impressions. These are all important skills in reading even though graphic representations of language seldom contain signals for intonation, stress, and pause. These must be learned through associated auditory and kinesthetic recall.

In a study of the importance of visual associative language experience and the development of focused attention, Mackworth (1973) emphasizes that reading basically involves the organization of visual symbols into a verbal code that has already acquired some meaning. Other work, such as that of Lundberg (1977), warns us that in some children (among them dyslexics) emphasis on the development of automatic auditory decoding may be overvalued and even detrimental. If a child has not yet developed focused attention and discrimination, overattention to auditory decoding will interfere with comprehension since true language functions cannot become automatic on a preattentive-discriminatory level. Similarly, Denckla (1977) recognizes the fundamental auditory processing problem of dyslexics and proposes that remedial techniques and procedures should stress visual-symbol learning, which is an easier first step for these children.

Although visual-symbol learning may be easier than auditory decoding for most dyslexic children, most of them have more visual processing deficiencies than nondyslexic children. Therefore, developmental and remedial programs continue to experiment with new ways to improve those visual-symbol processing skills that have been closely identified with learning to read. Spache (1976) presents a summary of seven training programs that emphasize visual discrimination and related processing skills. Almost all of these programs focus on the direct discrimination of letters, words, forms, and other symbolic material using prescriptive lessons, games, tachistoscopic presentations, and other visual training activities. All seven of the studies showed specific gains in those reading-readiness and visual-linguistic skills required for reading.

SYMBOL DISCRIMINATION

Some of the more important perceptual-linguistic symbol discrimination skills required for reading are:

- differentiating and explaining story pictures in children's picture books
- matching letter and number shapes
- matching words and word forms
- identifying reversals in symbol, letter, and word forms

- discriminating initial and final differences in words
- determining fine differences in words and symbols

Several experiments, such as those by Lyle and Goyen (1968) with retarded readers, demonstrate that reading-disabled children perform much worse than nondisabled readers on tasks requiring visual discrimination of letters, lines, and shapes under immediate, delayed, or sequential conditions. This deficiency was found to be in the visual decoding process itself. Earlier work by Goins (1958) demonstrates that poor readers of normal or superior intelligence lacked sufficient training in the visual perceptual analysis of words. This lack resulted in numerous reading errors. Witelson (1976) produces evidence of right-hemispheric spatial processing immaturity in young dyslexic boys and argues for emphasizing early visual-spatial discrimination training for such children.

Considerable evidence exists that visual processing skills can be developed through direct instruction. For example, Moyer and Newcomer (1977) review twelve major studies showing that the ability to detect letter-orientation relationships and to correct reversal errors is learned through direct training. Some of the more successful visual training tasks used in these studies included directional symbol matching, verbalization of letter discriminations, directional memory activity, and motor skill involvement.

Many of these findings have led to the creation of visual discrimination programs, workbooks, and kits for use with exceptional children. Some examples are listed below:

Peabody Language Development Kits (American Guidance Service), a series of four developmental language kits, stress the acquisition of oral language and visual processing skills. Each kit contains colorful picture cards and materials for analysis and discussion. Visual reception and convergent thinking are developed by sequential lessons. Research by Dunn (1967) shows significant acceleration in reading progress by underprivileged children using these materials.

Words in Color (Gattegno 1963) teaches letter discrimination, followed by letter sound sequences and word naming. Different colors are used for selected phonemes to aid in discrimination. (Similar uses of color to stress phonics, structure, or word analysis are presented by Trela (1968) and appear in several other systems.)

Visual Readiness Skills and **Visual Discrimination** (The Continental Press, Inc.) are a series of five liquid duplicator books of twenty-four lessons each. Almost all of the activities in these booklets use complex forms, letters, and words. Visual discrimination responses can be made by pointing or marking on the worksheet.

Rebus Reading Programs (American Guidance Service) use pictorial or symbolic representation to suggest words or syllables. A number of programs develop rebus picture vocabularies of more than one hundred words for introductory "picture reading." After picture reading the child is transferred to traditional written material (Woodcock 1968). This approach has also been modified for use with other kinds of handicapped children.

In an intensive reinforcement study using magnetic symbols and word cards, DeVilliers and Naughton (1974) taught autistic children to make sight word discriminations, to read simple sentences, and to generalize meanings. Such studies show that representational material can be used in developing visual processing skills and may contribute to total reading performance.

Three different lessons for the development of visual discrimination skills follow. It should be kept in mind that these lessons are only examples and should be modified to meet the needs of a particular student. They are representative of the kinds of learning tasks that have been found to be of value in the development of specific perceptual-linguistic processing skills.

SYMBOL TRACKING

As soon as children are able to make basic visual discriminations they begin to follow objects and symbols in space. With experience they acquire the ability to fixate on printed material, to hold it in focus, and to coordinate ocular movements. The following four visual tracking skills are essential for reading:

- determining picture story sequences in books and comics
- finding letters in symbol sequence
- following words and phrases
- scanning and locating directed words, sentences, and paragraphs

Objective: to match letters and symbols

Materials: worksheet and pencil

Directions: Mark the letter or symbol on the right of the page that is exactly like the one on the left.

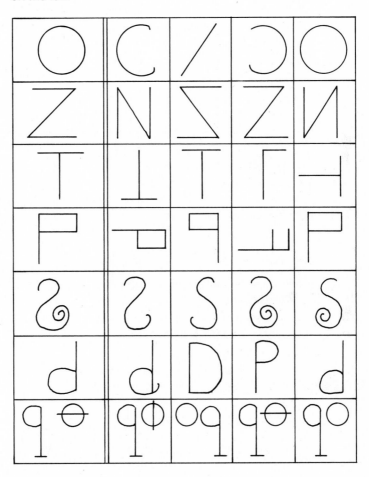

Evaluation: Number correct _____

                     Kind of error_____

Variations: Have the child correct errors by tracing the figure with his or her finger. Have children create their own symbols and worksheets.

Objective: to associate color with symbols and words

Materials: picture cards, colored felt pens, worksheet

Directions: A. Look at these pictures and tell me what they are:

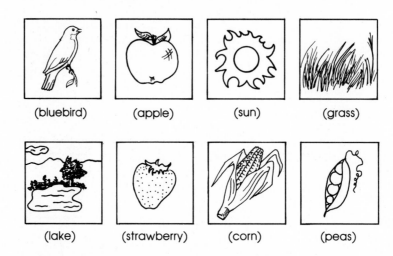

(bluebird)   (apple)   (sun)   (grass)

(lake)   (strawberry)   (corn)   (peas)

Use a blue felt pen to trace over the bluebird and the lake.

What color is an apple? Yes, it is usually red–trace the picture of the apple and the strawberry with a red pen.

What colors should we use for the other pictures? Yes, yellow for the sun and corn, and green for grass and peas.

Now I am writing the words for these pictures–you are to underline each word with the appropriate color and tell me what word you are underlining.

B. Here is the alphabet:

a b c d e f g h i j k l m n
o p q r s t u v w x y z

Place a red dot inside the letter **d.**
Place a green dot inside the letter **q.**

Evaluation: Number correct _____

Kinds of errors _____

Variations: Color vowels; trace easily reversed letters in different colors.

Objective: to discriminate fine differences in nonsense symbols

Materials: worksheet and red felt pen

Directions: Look at the word symbols below and place a red circle around the one on the right that looks like the one on the left.

O + $	O x $	O +$	O + S	O + &
manq	maup	menp	manq	maqu
Poat	boot	poat	Poat	doat
deeer	deere	deree	deaer	deeer
pipqp	pipqp	piqpp	pippq	piqqi
Threi	their	there	threi	Threi
ghist	ghsit	ghist	ghost	Ghist
Kriel	kreil	Kriel	keilr	krlie
shepe	sheqe	sheep	shepe	shgee
xtrop	xtrep	xtuoq	xtrpo	xtrop

Evaluation: Number correct _____

Kinds of errors _____

Variations: Use real words with two or three word sentence matching. Have children make up their own lists using a primary typewriter.

In his study of reading deficiencies and their remediation, Gray (1922) shows that both reading rate and comprehension are positively correlated with the length of perception span: older and better readers have fewer eye-movement pauses per line with shorter pauses and fewer regressive movements. This finding is confirmed by Goins (1958) and other investigators who advocate the use of visual tracking exercises, space markers, and mechanical pacing techniques to improve the efficient perception of visual stimuli.

Several studies, such as those by Sells and Fixott (1957), show that tachistoscopic training can enlarge the size of the visual form field, increase reading speed and comprehension, and improve the visual judgment of distance, angulation, and estimation of area. Other work by Leisman (1975) substantiates that saccadic eye movements of short duration and high velocity are also related to information summation problems and to difficulties in making critical judgments.

Visual processing training should involve fixation, integration, and interpretation of symbolic material that is meaningfully related to reading. A number of tracking and visual pursuit exercises for use by special educators have been created by Behrmann (1970). Some other widely used materials include:

The Michigan Tracking Program (Ann Arbor Publishers) is a series of excellent workbooks that develop symbol-tracking skills, such as the visual sequencing of objects, letters, and words. The workbook lessons are well organized and can be used by all age groups in prescriptive and self-instructional settings.

Visual Perceptual Skills Filmstrips (Educational Records Sales) is a series of developmental filmstrip exercises for classroom or clinical use that includes visual sequencing and tracking.

Zweig-Bruno Stereo-Tracing Exercise Program (Keystone View Company) is essentially a visual tracking program to strengthen the dominant eye using the stereo-reader device available from the same company. Materials may also be used for normal tracking using both eyes.

Following are three sample lessons to develop tracking ability.

Objective: to follow with one's eyes a path that leads to a target

Materials: tracking cards or sheets

Directions: Look at each of the cards below. Follow each of the symbols on the left with your eyes and tell me what it leads to.

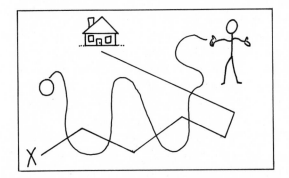

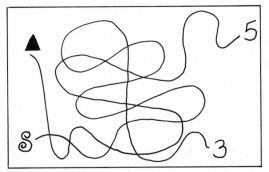

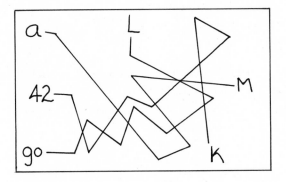

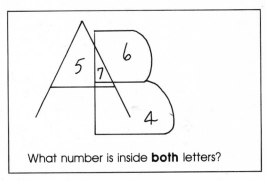

What number is inside **both** letters?

Evaluation:

Card	Time	+	-
1			
2			
3			
4			

Variations: Use action words at the end of the track, such as "jump," "smile," "clap," and have the child act out the word.

Objective: to coordinate one's eyes to select designated letters

Materials: worksheet and pencil

Directions: Look at the alphabet letters in the box below:

Box A

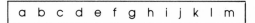

a b c d e f g h i j k l m

Put a circle around the letter **a** in the box and then circle the first **a** that you see in box B below. Then put a circle around the letter **b** in the box and the first **b** below. Do the same with all the letters being sure to circle only the first letter that you see.

Box B

Tncdkat! fhtiopoklm neu ksy jbx it.

qir mibjo trio mon rescrit of ripd pm.

xtgot oto rip, op.

In box C below circle **all** of the letter **a**'s that you see. Then draw a line through **all** of the letter **m**'s that you see.

Box C

This is the time of the year when everyone begins to think of Christmas. The snow is gently falling and the weather is crisp. I am looking forward to decorating the tree!

Evaluation:

	Time required (min./sec.)	Number of errors
A		
B		

Variations: Use the rest of the letters of the alphabet. Have students make extended sentences and paragraphs.

Objective: to locate words in sentences

Materials: workcards and colored pen

Directions: Look at the cards with the underlined words. Circle the first word that is under-
                      lined in red and then find that word on the next line and circle it. Then circle
                      the second word that is underlined and find it on the line below. Do the same
                      for the other words that are underlined.

Card A

dogs chase cats			
digs	dogs	dirt	dark
chose	chit	chase	cheese
cats	cows	cars	cuts

Card B

do you like ice cream?				
to	do	bo	de	dot
your	you	you're	yard	year
lick	like	look	lark	lid
ice	is	it	lice	ick
cram	cream	creep	crip	crop

Evaluation:

Card	Time	Errors
A		
B		

Variations: Use window "place-marking cards" to reduce distractions in locating words
                      and phrases in more complex paragraphs.

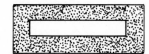

VISUAL ORGANIZATION

When children can discriminate, sequence, and integrate symbols, they have acquired visual organization. The key perceptual-linguistic aspect of visual organization is *meaningful* integration of symbolic material with other sensory data. A few of the more important visual organization skills in reading are:

- completing incomplete letters and words
- matching upper and lowercase words
- adding letters or symbols
- deleting letters or symbols
- substituting letters or symbols
- relating word symbols to other similar word symbols

In a summary of research on reading processes, Venezky (1977) reports on experiments of Cattell and others showing the importance of gestalt organization and meaning in reading. Experimental subjects required twice as much time to read unconnected words aloud as words connected in sentences, and the perceptual span for letters in meaningful words was considerably greater than for letters in random strings. Visual organization training should therefore involve meaningful material as much as possible.

The extensive work of Wiig and Semel (1976) further supports a gestalt approach to remediation. Efficient reading has been shown to depend on semantic rules of language, and written material is processed in terms of meaningful phrase units based on structure and content (and not just word-by-word). Since reading comprehension is a function of similarity between language structure patterns in written materials and the child's oral language, dyslexia involves semantic and word substitution problems as well as visual symbol confusion and problems in grapheme-phoneme association. Wiig and Semel advocate a number of excellent cognitive processing remedial tasks including the visual organization of spatial-temporal-sequential relationships. They propose still other semantic organization activities for the comprehension of verbs, adjectives, pronouns, prepositions, antonyms, synonyms, homonyms, multiple-meaning words, verbal analogies, comparative relationships, idioms, and proverbs.

However, on a more fundamental level of visual organization training many different sensory-motor manipulative activities should be involved since organization and integration are furthered through the use of materials that can be arranged in space and time. Kaluger and Kolson (1969) advocate the use of kinesthetic touch lessons to further visual organization and left-hemispheric development. Suggested lessons include form-symbol discrimination, color cues, and music and rhythmic games, together with the Kolson-Kaluger method of using the Keystone stereo-reader. In practice, most children with severe reading problems have varied kinds of visual organization-integrative disabilities. In one clinical study by Swanson (1971–1972) of one hundred random patients in visual training, 78 percent demonstrated visual integrative dysfunctions (73 percent were dyslexic and 43 percent had strephosymbolia). Prescriptive remediation required the development of several related visual skills.

Some very important research has been done on visual asymmetry and reading proficiency. As we have already discussed in Chapter 2, there is lateralization of brain hemispheric functions. In the visual system, there is a cross-over of retinal neural fibers so that controlled stimulation of left or right visual halffields is selectively processed to the left or right hemisphere. For example, tachistoscopically presented words to either the left or right visual fields can be systematically programmed. Symbolic sight-word identification primarily requiring simple visual-spatial analysis is largely a right (nondominant) brain function while complex word analysis, association, and linguistic interpretation occurs in the left (dominant) hemisphere where visual-auditory integration takes place.

Several researchers, such as Miller and Turner (1973) and Bakker (1977), have experimented with elementary-school children in different grades using simultaneous tachistoscopic presentation of simple words to both left and right visual fields. Right field (left hemispheric) superiority did not develop until children were in the fourth grade or beyond. The implication is that visual organization training is an important right-hemispheric function that appears to be underdeveloped in dyslexic children and requires special training (Witelson 1976).

Visual organization training and development is best conducted with multisensory lessons and materials such as those listed below. However, recent experiments with tachistoscopic and stereo-reader lateral-development programs may lead to techniques for the direct programming of the right-hemispheric visual area in young dyslexic children. At this time however, most classroom and clinical training involves the simultaneous use of both eyes in the systematic organization and integration of symbolic visual material. Training materials commonly used in this area include the following:

GOAL Language Development Programs (Milton Bradley Company) are packaged kits based on the ITPA model. Lesson cards and materials include numerous learning activities for developing visual association, visual closure, visual reception, and related psycholinguistic skills.

The Frostig Program for the Development of Visual Perception (Follett Corporation) contains a series of developmental workbooks and materials that can be used to teach spatial relationship and visual organization skills. It must be extended and supplemented, though, with the addition of more symbolic material such as letters and words.

Developing Visual Awareness and Insight (Instructional Materials and Equipment Distributors) is a useful workbook containing many different kinds of visual organization activities. This is best used as introductory training for the *Phonic Series* books, by the same company, for developing word recognition.

Developing Learning Readiness (Webster Division, McGraw-Hill Book Company) is a kit containing six programs for young children. It includes eye movement charts and filmstrips of symbolic material helpful in the development of visual organization skills.

Spatial Organization Workbooks I, II, III: The Fitzhugh Plus Program (Allied Education Council) are self-instructional materials specially developed for use with persons who have cerebral dysfunction and learning deficiencies. Visual organization tasks proceed from simple form discrimination through the organization and integration of advanced figural relationships and word symbols. Especially valuable for older children and adolescents.

Following are sample exercises in visual organization.

Objective: to organize and interpret visual symbols verbally

Materials: worksheet, ink, or water colors

Directions: Look at the ink blot below. Try to imagine some objects or symbols that the ink blot suggests to you. Tell me what you can see.

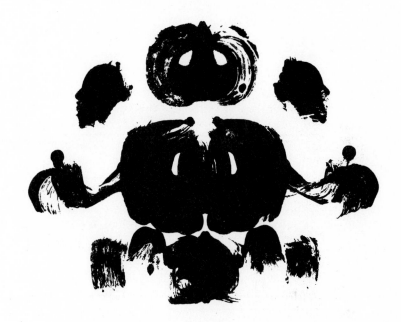

Take a sheet of white paper and paint. With your brush dab some different colors on the paper, fold it over in the middle and press both sides together. Now unfold the paper and tell me as many different things as you can imagine.

Evaluation:

	Number of objects perceived	Verbal expression		
		+	+ /-	-
A				
B				

Variations: Have children record their verbal descriptions on tape recorders. Play back and evaluate.

Objective: to complete, organize, and interpret letters and words visually

Materials: worksheet

Directions: Point to each symbol below, visually fill in the missing parts and then tell me what the completed symbol is and what it means.

1. 1 8 A F 7 9 0

2. 2 0 5 L N S Z

3.
boy	girl	man	woman
b__y	gi__l	ma__	w__m__n

4.
I go to school
I g__ to s__hool

5.
man	doll	apple	rain
ap__le	r__in	do__l	m__n

6.
fish	wagon	puppy	stick	kitten	window
wag__n	stic__	kit__en	f__sh	w__nd__w	

7.
o i u	The d__g bites

8.
a e i o u	A c__w gives m__lk

Evaluation: Number correct _____

Kinds of errors _____

Variations: Have children make up their own incomplete letters and words. Combine with visual-motor tracing and copying activities.

VISUAL MEMORY

The retention of learned visual symbols such as letters, words, and punctuation marks is an important aspect of the reading process. Training most often begins with direct visual matching and recall of designs and symbols. Later a child must be able to recall and reproduce visual sequences of printed material after a delay of several days or more. Four important developmental visual-memory skills are:

- recalling picture story sequences
- recalling design and nonsense word patterns
- recalling letter and digit sequences
- recalling syllables, words, and phrases

Research shows that significant visual memory deficiencies are common in dyslexic children. A study by Rizzo (1939) was one of the earliest to establish the relationship between poor visual memory and reading retardation. Later, Kass (1963) found visual sequential memory deficiencies a reliable indicator in identifying children with reading disabilities. A study of factors involved in the early identification of specific language and reading disabilities by Oliphant (1969) further confirms the primary importance of visual memory and demonstrates the value of the visual memory subtests (subtests 3 and 5) on the Slingerland screening tests for this purpose: the subtest 3 correlation with the Stanford Achievement Test total reading score was $r = -.46$ while subtest 5 had a $r = -.44$.

A review of the research on visual memory for letters, letter clusters, and sight words by Groff (1974) concludes that children learn to read most effectively by first learning to use letters and letter clusters as cues to word recognition. He suggests that visual discrimination of letters be taught using kinesthetic techniques followed by phonic training. In a similar study of information-processing deficiencies and reading disability by Morrison, Giordani, and Nagy (1977), highly significant memory problems were found in poor readers with particularly severe symbolic deficiencies in encoding and organizational retrieval (using tachistoscopic recall of geometric forms, letters, and abstract designs). However, Rudel, Denckla, and Spalten (1976) conducted paired associate learning of Morse code and Braille letters with dyslexic and nondyslexic children and conclude that visual symbols are more quickly learned than auditory ones by reading-disabled boys, and that this kind of initial visual learning should be used and strongly reinforced.

Halliwell and Solan (1972) studied 105 first-grade children in three experimental groups and compared them with a control group of 35 children. The six-month training program stressed intensive tachistoscopic exposure and memory training tasks together with other perceptual-learning activities and regular remedial reading instruction. The criterion measure was improvement on the Reading Comprehension Subtest of the Metropolitan Achievement Test. The most significant gains were made by boys whose initial test scores were low. The results indicate a need for further development of these critical readiness skills.

In another study, Boucher (1976) conducted an experiment on the effects of specific memory training on reading achievement. Using learning-disabled children, she carried out a visual and auditory memory training program for forty-five minutes a day over a twelve-week period. Visual training covered discrimination and recall of pictures, objects, shapes, letters, words, and ideas using tachistoscopes, flashcards, and other materials. A twelve-step memory-training program was carefully designed and included the following units:

1. form perception
2. visual memory for forms
3. visual memory for sequences of forms
4. visual and auditory memory for directions
5. perception of letters
6. visual memory for letters
7. auditory memory for letters
8. visual and auditory sequencing of letter sounds
9. visual-auditory memory for vowels
10. visual-auditory memory for digraphs and diphthongs
11. two rules for changing vowel sounds
12. word parts and rhymes

Boucher's program also included a systematic reinforcement system using both tokens and praise. Significant improvement at the .05 level was noted on the Comprehensive Test of Basic Skills (reading test), the Slingerland visual and auditory memory subtests, the ITPA visual and auditory sequential memory subtests, and the Bender Visual-Motor Gestalt (memory) test. The greatest gain from this program was an 81 percent reduction of errors on the Slingerland visual memory tasks.

Again, it can be readily seen that almost all visual memory training programs involve the use of other modalities. All such programs require at least minimal responses such as pointing and some verbalization, and some require the use of all the senses. Useful visual-memory training materials for teachers and clinicians include:

Design Sequence Cards and **Visual Word Perception Cards** (Academic Therapy Publications) are sets of progressively more difficult designs and words used to develop visual memory and sequencing skills.

Visual Language Materials (Newby Visual Language, Inc.) is a useful series of picture-sequence cards and workbooks for the teaching of verbs, adjectives, pronouns, prepositions, and idioms.

Functional Word Recognition (Mast Development Company) includes five thousand frames in eight programmed Mast Cartridges to teach initial sight reading. Words have been selected from lists common to most basal reading series.

Dolch Basic Sight Word Materials (Garrard Publishing Company) are published by a company that produces a series of multisensory games and activities for helping children to acquire a sight vocabulary of 220 basic words and the most common nouns (Dolch 1960).

System 80 (Borg-Warner Educational Systems) is an outstanding audio-visual learning system for providing individualized instruction. A large visual console displays colorful and well-designed pictorial and symbolic learning tasks. The student listens to auditory directions, makes visual discriminations, and selects the answer by pushing a button. Feedback directs the child in making the proper choice. Curriculum materials are structured and nonconsumable. This system has been widely and successfully used in many special education programs.

Following are some examples of exercises to stimulate visual memory.

Objective: to place in sequence a series of visual symbols

Materials: symbol cards, worksheets

Directions: Look carefully at the symbols on the flashcards that I am about to show you. I will then turn the card over and you are to underline the correct symbol sequence on your worksheet.

1. [O $ A]	1. $ O A O $ A A $ O
2. [+ D5]	2. + D5 XD5 5Dº
3. [9T$b]	3. 9$Tb dT$b 9T$b
4. [CaYq]	4. CaYq CaYp CaYg
5. [Thik O]	5. thik O thiko Thik O
6. [Ya bit]	6. Ya bit ya bit yabit Yab it
7. [rock et]	7. Rock et rack et rock et
8. [oi ale ly]	8. oi ala ly oi ale ly oe lae ly oi ali ly
9. [a bare hare]	9. a hare bare a bare hare
	a bare pare a dare baer

Evaluation: Number correct _____

              Kinds of errors _____

Variations: Have the student draw single symbols on file cards for card sequencing. Use meaningful words and sentences from basal readers.

Objective: to recall symbol and letter sequences

Materials: worksheet

Directions: Look at the symbols on the worksheet and tell me which ones are missing from the blank spaces.

1. 5   6 __   8   9
2. 1   2 __   4   5 __   7   8
3. A __   C __   E __   G
4. GHI__   KLM__   PQR__
5. 1   3   5 __   2   4   6 __   5   7   9 __
6. __   B   C   __   f   g   __   u   v

7.   =   b __   y

8.   =   b   a __   l

9.   =   d __   g

10. 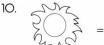   =   s __   n

Evaluation: Number correct _____

                    Kinds of errors _____

Variations: Use individual symbol cards so the student can arrange and manipulate sequences. Sequence short sentences.

Objective: to recall and verbally identify basic sight words and interpret their meaning

Materials: flashcards and worksheet

Directions: Look carefully at the word on the flashcard I show you. I will turn the flashcard over and you are to underline the correct word on your worksheet. Then, tell me the word and use it in a sentence.

1.	am	
2.	big	
3.	car	
4.	down	
5.	every	
6.	father	
7.	garden	
8.	horse	
9.	it is in	
10.	jump in	

Sight Word Worksheet

1.	an	as	am	at	
2.	but	buy	big	bed	box
3.	cap	cat	can	car	cow
4.	don't	draw	done	does	down
5.	eat	every	eggs	eight	
6.	found	farm	father	funny	
7.	grass	garden	going	green	
8.	horse	house	head	hand	hurt
9.	if it is	it is in	it is on		
10.	just in	just on	jump on	jump in	

Evaluation: Number correct _____

Words missed _____

Kinds of errors _____

Variations: Use the remainder of the Dolch list to make up other exercises. Use lists of words missed from current basal reader.

SUMMARY   The development of basic visual skills and the remediation of visual processing deficiencies are of concern to all specialists working with dyslexic children. Research and applied programs on symbol discrimination, symbol tracking, visual organization, and visual memory have been reviewed and illustrated. The effective development of visual skills always includes concomitant auditory, linguistic, and sensory-motor training.

Studies by Muehl and King (1967), among others, establish the significance of developing visual-processing skills for beginning reading. The most effective visual-training skill sequence for reading appears to be:

- matching letters
- matching words
- letter discrimination and naming
- letter sound association
- discriminating word forms in context

Children learn words best when meaning is emphasized by establishing associations with visual perceptions, words, sounds, and pictures. Other researchers such as Roswell and Natchez (1977) have developed a sequence of word-analysis skills for remedial education that begins with sight-word instruction (for example, the 95 most common nouns and the 220 basic sight words listed by Dolch). Specific auditory training should accompany prescriptive education for visual processing deficiencies.

DISCUSSION QUESTIONS AND ACTIVITIES

1. How might language-experience activities help shape visual processing skills?

2. List and define the major visual processing skills.

3. Discuss the development of visual processing skills as a compensatory approach for dyslexic children.

4. Demonstrate the use of the Continental Press duplicator book lessons (Visual Readiness Skills and Visual Discrimination).

5. Write a review of Behrmann's booklet *Activities for Developing Visual Perception.*

6. Use several of the sample lessons presented in this chapter with a reading-disabled student and evaluate the results.

7. Demonstrate the use of Keystone stereo-reader and discuss its use in the development of laterality.

8. How could visual-spatial organization activities be used to develop a recognition and understanding of verbs.

9. Write a paper discussing research on the Frostig Program for the Development of Visual Perception.

10. How are the Slingerland visual memory subtests related to reading?

11. Develop a diagnostic-prescriptive visual-memory lesson for a dyslexic child whose needs you know.

12. List several different mechanical devices, teaching machines, or special equipment that can be used to help develop visual processing skills in dyslexic children.

CHAPTER EIGHT

Remediating Auditory Processing Deficiencies

The process we call "seeing" involves the central nervous system in the integration of retinal impressions in the eye and their association with other perceptual data. The same is true for "hearing"—the ear is merely a receptor of sound waves requiring neuropsychological organization and interpretation in the brain. Functional hearing is a complex process requiring attention, reception, discrimination, association, and recall, all of which must then be meaningfully interrelated.

In reading the process is much more complicated. Reading demands the integration of both visual and auditory processing skills. This process culminates in a synthesis of phonemes and graphemes in a meaningful context. Accordingly, many investigators, such as Orton (1937), Wiig and Semel (1976), and Spache (1976a), stress the importance of developing basic auditory processing skills and remediating auditory deficiencies in children with severe reading disorders. In Chapter 2 of this book, we reviewed some of the research on significant auditory processing-skill differences between dyslexic and nondyslexic children. The most notable deficiencies requiring remediation involve the inability to sequence and synthesize sounds and letters into comprehensible patterns of words and phrases.

As studies reported by Venezky (1976, p. 166) show, "All rational approaches to reading instruction include both sight-word learning and letter-sound learning with its concomitant reliance on sound blending." But most developmental and remedial programs begin with the diagnostic evaluation and programming of the more basic auditory skills, which are prerequisites to higher-order reading processes. We will consider these important auditory processing skills in the four categories of auditory reception, auditory decoding, auditory memory, and auditory-vocal synthesis.

AUDITORY RECEPTION

Perhaps the most basic auditory skill is the ability to receive sound stimuli. Many things, such as severe ear infections, may result in blockage of sound waves and loss or distortion of hearing. Other forms of disease or injury to the auditory centers of the brain can result in central nervous system dysfunctions that disturb or distort neural impulses from sound waves. Many cases of auditory reception dysfunction are treated primarily by medical and audiological means, such as drugs, surgery, hearing aids, and special amplification devices.

In addition, the child with central nervous system processing and organization problems needs special education and training. In the more obvious cases of deaf and hard-of-hearing children, this kind of education has long been available. But it is only recently that prescriptive auditory-processing training has been made available to children with receptive aphasia or dyslexia. In fact, the recognition of auditory processing dysfunctions in learning-handicapped children whose impairment *is not* primarily a loss of acuity is fairly recent. The American Academy of Ophthalmology and Otolaryngology (1960) uses the term *dysacusis* to signify a dysfunction of the nervous system, the auditory nerve, or the cochlea that results in hearing loss and language problems. Studies by Myklebust (1954) establish the existence of several central nervous system communication disorders, such as auditory agnosia and imperception, that can culminate in both oral language and reading problems.

A few experimental remedial programs have been reported. Most of these studies conclude that creating an appropriate predisposition or "set" for reading is an intrinsic aspect of good auditory reception development programs. Carpenter (1972) reports an interesting case study of an auditory dyslexic. The study underscores the importance of developing basic processing skills. Spache (1976b, pp. 417–418) summarizes twelve apparently successful perceptual training programs for reading-disabled children that stressed receptivity for cognitive learning. Most of these programs were multisensory approaches, but two had auditory training components that resulted in readiness gains and improved reading performance. Almost all good auditory reception programs require systematic visual-auditory-verbal integration approaches. Such an approach, described by Forrest (1972), resulted in an increase in focused attention and subsequent achievement. Some instructional materials are listed below.

Binaural Auditory Trainers (AMBCO Electronics) are useful since many dyslexic children can profit from sound amplification and discrimination training. Binaural auditory trainers can be obtained in portable and stationary models. Earphones can be controlled to produce the desired reception in either ear.

Phonic Mirror (H. C. Electronics, Inc.) is an automatic speech playback recorder that can give controlled playback or continuously repeat recorded stimuli. Auditory attention, reception, and discrimination are all enhanced through use of the immediate feedback provided by such machines.

Rhyming—Levels A,B,C, (Continental Press, Inc.) are three workbooks, typical of the better materials available, that progress from simple to complex learning tasks. Rhyming activities and programs should be an intrinsic part of auditory-temporal receptivity training.

Visual Echo II (Visual Echo Company) is an example of devices that combine visual and auditory training. This instrument responds to sound stimuli such as words, syllables, and phrase reading with a colored light display (visual feedback).

Following are examples of auditory reception exercises.

Objective: to learn to listen more carefully and to increase left-hemispheric auditory receptivity

Materials: binaural auditory trainer, stereophonic headphones, blindfold, tape recorder

Directions: Listen carefully to the sounds you are about to hear. When you no longer hear the sounds, turn on the tape recorder and reproduce the sounds exactly as you heard them. Your left earphone should be turned off.

1. • Here is a small drum and beater. Turn on the tape recorder, beat a pattern on the drum, then replay your recording. Now repeat the pattern you heard on the tape.
   • This time we have two drums and beaters. First, I will play a slow beat like this. Now turn on the recorder and join me in playing the pattern together.
   • Now you create a slow but different beat and I will attempt to repeat it as we record it.

2. Now I am blindfolding you. Listen carefully to what you hear as we will record and play back your response: (Sounds: clapping hands, coughing, tearing paper, closing a book, "meow," "woof, woof," "moo, moo," "happy birthday," "Mike, bike, like," Harry, Mary, Larry")

3. You are still blindfolded. Listen carefully and do what I tell you to do: touch your nose, stand up, scratch your right ear.

Evaluation: Number correct _____

Kinds of errors _____

Variations: Repeat exercises using left earphone only. Increase amplification. Use reading tasks.

Objective: to discriminate, duplicate, and associate rhyming words and concepts

Materials: worksheet and pencil

Directions: 1. Listen to the first word I say and hold up your hand when you hear another
                      word that rhymes with it:

         star: horse, **car**, man
         deer: **ear**, button, pear
         clock: dog, **lock**, drum, ship
         lamb: wood, **ham**, hands, **dam**
         moon: tire, shave, **spoon**

2. Listen to the first word I say and repeat it after me. Then listen to all of the
   words that follow and tell me the one word that rhymes with the first word:

         ships: **hips**, comb, whip
         bank: lake, beat, **tank**
         thumb: lamb, **drum**, ski, box
         chief: bone, **beef**, bat, bird
         pool: hail, bale, **school**, tale

3. Listen to the riddles and the three possible answers to them and tell me the
   correct answer:

    • I rhyme with **bed** and I am a color (head, **red**, dead).
    • I rhyme with **blue** and you can wear me (moo, glue, **shoe**).
    • I rhyme with **comb** and people live inside of me (foam, **home**, roam).
    • I rhyme with trailer and I work on a ship (bailer, **sailor**, layer, player).

4. Listen to the riddles and tell me the answer that rhymes:

    • I rhyme with **now** and I live on a farm.
    • I rhyme with **joke** and I go up chimneys.
    • I rhyme with **light** and children fly me in the sky.

Evaluation:

Tasks	Number Correct	Kinds of Errors
1		
2		
3		

Variations: Have children create their own rhymes and riddles. Use nursery rhymes with
                      missing words.

AUDITORY DECODING

Auditory decoding may be defined as discriminating fine sounds and associating them so that they make sense. When children decode they are trying to give meaning to the many sounds they have heard.

Children learn to decode by directing their attention to the patterned cues being presented to them. Through careful listening, directed focus and attention, practice, and reinforcement, they gradually begin to refine and organize their auditory perceptions. With reading, auditory decoding is part of a more complex visual-auditory associative process in which sounds are cued and coded with written symbols.

Several studies have been made on the training of children in auditory decoding skills. Rohr (1968) conducted an extensive perceptual program that included training in identifying hidden noises, distinguishing consonant blends, and duplicating monosyllables and musical patterns on a xylophone. The most successful activity was having a child listen to a tape recording and simultaneously to a story read by the teacher. The child was instructed to attend to just one auditory source and later to answer questions about that source. Children trained in this way improved in reading and increased their attention spans.

In a doctoral study of the effects of auditory-perceptual training on the performance of second graders, Semel (1972) found significant auditory gains as a result of systematic instruction. Hammill and Larsen (1974) critically review the research and conclude that much of the time devoted to auditory training needs to be carefully reevaluated to ensure it is task relevant to the reading process (if the objective is to improve reading performance). An example of relevant training is given by Durrell and Murphy (1958) who found that, because of training, children with auditory discrimination deficiencies made significant gains in auditory word analysis. In another relevant experiment Zedler (1969) stressed oral language, phonics, sentence patterning, and the development of auditory comprehension by reading special material aloud. Zedler reports that an experimental group made twice the gains of a control group.

Venezky (1976) discusses an experimental five-year program with kindergarten children in several states. The program emphasized training in decoding skills that were basically attentional and informational, such as matching sound with words and identifying sounds and syllables within words. Significant improvement in an experimental group was noted in both reading performance and attitude toward learning.

Other auditory decoding programs have resulted in promising instructional techniques for use in prescriptive education. Kaluger and Kolson (1969, pp. 225-226) stress the importance of rhythm techniques and recommend the following training sequence as a part of a total remedial approach:

- repeating short sentences perfectly
- learning and saying jingles and rhymes
- listening to and obeying commands
- marching and dancing to simple rhythms
- scribbling or finger painting in time to rhythms
- singing rhythmical songs and action songs
- following a sequence of directions
- sound blending

Research by Tallal (1976) on dyslexics shows that these children can process and decode difficult auditory information, but at a much slower rate than nondyslexic children. Tallal's work also raises the interesting possibility that right-ear training for auditory temporal processing might be necessary for stimulating development of the main language centers of the left hemisphere. Perhaps differential aural stimulation to the right ear, such as the use of different words, sentences, and frequencies (whispering or shouting), might enhance auditory decoding skills in dyslexics.

A few of the major auditory decoding training materials available for use by special educators follow:

The Auditory Discrimination in Depth Program—ADD (Teaching Resources Corporation) is designed to make children aware of the sound structure of language and have them discriminate speech sounds and determine sound sequences and patterns as in syllables and words. The student uses colored blocks to give some concrete reality to the development of sound-symbol associations. The final goal of the program is development of facility in spelling and reading. One study by Lindamood (1967) reports that an experimental group of thirty-six children selected for study with ADD made appreciable gains in oral reading and in auditory conceptualization.

Developing Auditory Awareness and Insight (Instructional Materials and Equipment Distributors) is a teacher's handbook by Selma Herr that contains a number of stimulating activities for developing auditory decoding skills. It is best used along with other books in this series on perceptual communication skills.

Semel Auditory Processing Programs (Follett Publishing Company) is a series of "sound-order-sense" lessons for young children. In these lessons students judge whether certain language sequences make sense. Wiig and Semel (1973) modified this program and report significant improvement in the comprehension of linguistic concepts and logical-processing deficiciencies.

Some sample auditory decoding exercises follow.

AUDITORY MEMORY

The ability to retain and organize sounds is essential in reading. Sequential sound organization and patterning is a difficult skill for dyslexic children to acquire. A study by Golden and Steiner (1969) shows that among second-grade children good readers are significantly superior to poor readers on both the sound blending and the auditory sequential memory subtests of the ITPA. Many other studies, such as those by Bryden (1972), Ealck (1973), Spring (1976), and Badian (1977), confirm the existence of significant auditory memory deficiencies in dyslexic and other children with severe reading disabilities. Practically all research results support prescriptive intervention for the remediation of auditory memory deficiencies in these children.

A number of different techniques and programs have been devised to develop auditory memory skills. One of the most direct approaches to reading is the Initial Teaching Alphabet (i.t.a.). It consists of only forty-four visual-sound symbols and reduces the auditory-visual memory problem for dyslexic children. The i.t.a. program is normally introduced to first-grade children who learn and remember consistent sound patterns. Studies by Downing (1965) and Lane (1974) report on the general effectiveness of i.t.a. lessons. Research by Gardner (1966) in a six-month remedial-reading program establishes the superiority of i.t.a. over traditional lessons with primary-grade reading-disabled children. Lane's research shows that i.t.a. can achieve

Objective: to discriminate fine differences between spoken words and to associate them with manuscript letters.

Materials: worksheet

Directions: Listen carefully to the words and sounds I say. When I am through you say the words and sounds. Then, if they are exactly alike you say "yes." If they are not alike say "no."

1. girl – girl	16. V – B
2. man – ban	17. lock – lock
3. ah – ah	18. rock – rock
4. D – E	19. lock – clock
5. fist – fist	20. shoe – zoo
6. goat – boat	21. cat – cat
7. eyes – eyes	22. bat – hat
8. B – D	23. mat – mat
9. A – A	24. chain – chain
10. grass – glass	25. C – E
11. mouse – mouth	26. clown – brown
12. fan – fan	27. plane – cane
13. watch – wash	28. train – train
14. coat – coat	29. show – blue
15. face – vase	30. cap – cap

Evaluation: Circle the number for each correct answer. Write in specific errors made for each sound pair.

Variations: Place alphabet cards in the chalkboard tray. Have the student pick the initial consonants in the words he or she says. Have the student define words that are different and explain how and why they sound different.

Objective: to think of and verbalize words that "go together" logically

Materials: worksheet, alphabet cards

Directions:

1. You will find baseballs and bats in a sports store. Tell me as many other things that you can think of that might also be found in a sports store.

2. Tell me all the things you might find in a large grocery store.

3. This time take each letter of the alphabet in order and tell me a food that starts with that sound. For example, a = apple, b = beets, c = carrots, and so forth.

4. Here is a pack of alphabet cards for you to spread out on the table. Select five of the cards and place them in front of you. Pick up one card at a time and tell me three different words that begin with that letter sound.

5. Listen to the mixed-up words I will say. When I have finished you are to unscramble them and reorganize the words into a sensible order.

   - man / a   (a man)
   - the / dog / big   (the big dog)
   - 1 2 3 8 5 6 7 4   (1 2 3 4 5 6 7 8)
   - A B H D E F G C   (A B C D E F G H)
   - December / Christmas / is / in   (Christmas is in December)

Evaluation:

Task	Number correct	Kinds of errors
1		
2		
3		
4		
5		

Variations: Play word association games with the children taking turns. For children already reading, use word cards of food and other objects. Have the child pick out the card that matches his or her answer.

Objective: to understand and use parts of the Morse code

Materials: international Morse code cards, electric buzzer board

Directions:

1. Look at the Morse code cards arranged on your desk. When put together the letters spell the word **man**:

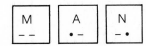

Each letter has a special sound of dots and dashes. Listen to the buzzer board make the dots and dashes for the word **man**. Now I will make the sounds for each letter again and as I do so you hand me the correct letter card.

2. Look at the Morse code cards below:

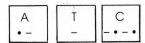

Now listen to the sounds I make on the buzzer board and then put that letter in front of you. Here is the first one (C), here is the next one (A), and here is the last one (T). What are the three letters? Together they spell **cat**–say **cat**.

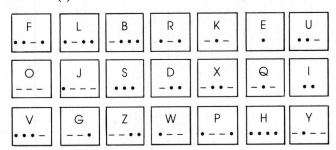

4. Now rearrange all of the cards in alphabetical order and then pick out the letters in your first name and place them in front of you. Listen carefully now as I buzz out the letters; after I buzz the letter you hand me that card.

5. Tell me three words to buzz out in Morse code. Now let us find the letters for each word. This time you buzz out each letter and say the letter.

Evaluation: Number correct _____

Kinds of errors _____

Variations: Have the child buzz a code for teacher to decode.

good results with sixth-grade reading disabled children. For many dyslexic children, the i.t.a. approach simplifies difficult auditory-memory processing tasks such as recalling proper letter-sound associations and is therefore a valuable beginning instructional strategy.

Other special methods have been used and found helpful in training auditory memory skills. For example, an "auditory-vocal activation" method devised by Kaliski (1977) for use with language-disabled children stresses the development of auditory memory skills through the use of singing, piano playing, and related rhythmic activities. Another program developed by Boucher (1976) integrates sequential memory-training lessons with other program components. Boucher reports significant gains on the auditory memory subtest of the ITPA, the auditory subtest of the Slingerland Screening Test, and the reading subtest of the Comprehensive Test of Basic Skills.

Similarly, Zovko (1977) describes a diagnostic-prescriptive approach to the auditory training of dyslexic children that progresses from auditory recall and synthesis of one-syllable words to words of two or more syllables, and from familiar words to less frequently used words. Zovko and her colleagues at the Suvag Center for the Rehabilitation of Speech and Hearing in Zagreb, Yugoslavia, use a special electronic machine, the Suvag Lingue, which facilitates the selection of an optimal frequency field for words and stimulates the development of aural perception. This machine is equipped with a special sound vibrator, which the child can place on his or her wrist, forehead, knee, and other body locations to feel the sound feedback from syllables being pronounced.

Some instructional materials that develop auditory memory skills are listed below:

Auditory Perception Training Programs (Developmental Learning Materials) include a training kit of five programs dealing with auditory memory, auditory discrimination, auditory figure-ground, auditory motor, and auditory imagery. The auditory memory program has cassette tapes and spirit-duplicating master worksheets that serve as visual representation response sheets to taped auditory stimuli.

Initial Teaching Alphabet Reading Program (Fearon Pitman Publishers, Inc.) is a highly systematic decoding program with a series of readers, workbooks, and sound-symbol cards. The program develops basic word analysis and consistent sound-symbol associations for acquiring a 650-word vocabulary.

Special Language Audio Flashcard Program (Electronic Futures, Inc.) is a series of ninety ten-minute lessons for developing basic language patterns, following simple directions, and acquiring related skills. Sets of sound-taped flashcards are used with the mechanical audio flashcard reader. This program can be used as auditory memory training preliminary to the more advanced reading flashcard series.

Examples of auditory memory exercises follow.

AUDITORY-VOCAL SYNTHESIS

The most important auditory processing skill in reading (and the most difficult one for dyslexic children to learn) is auditory-vocal synthesis. This complex skill requires the integration of visual letter symbols (graphemes) with their corresponding sounds (phonemes) in a vocal sequence that has meaning. Luria (1966) and other neuropsychologists have demonstrated that difficulties in phonetic analysis and synthesis (such as blending) may result from dysfunction in the auditory cortex. This dysfunction usually requires compensatory training with intensive multisensory/kinesthetic remedial techniques.

Considerable research has established that phonic skills are essential for reading. In her classic study on learning to read, Chall (1967, p. 150) discusses the results of seventeen major investigations on predictive reading abilities. The investigations showed that in the primary grades "knowing the sound values of the letters and being able to hear similarities and differences in the spoken words have greater influence on reading achievement" than mental ability or other predictive measures. In a review of thirty-three studies on selected auditory perceptual skills and reading ability, Hammill and Larsen (1974) found that in the primary grades both phonemic-discrimination and sound-blending skills had positive correlation with word recognition although sound blending was even more significant in grades 7 through 12. Sound blending in first grade was also found to predict silent-reading ability in the third grade.

Spache's (1976a) research on phonics shows that emphasizing isolated letter sounds tends to produce stronger ability to name words. He also discovered that overemphasis of phonic systems tends to devalue meaning and leads to poor scores on tests of comprehension, especially among pupils of lower mental ability. An extensive report by

AUDITORY MEMORY LESSON   REMEMBERING SEQUENTIAL INFORMATION

Objective: to recall meaningful words in proper order

Materials: alphabet cards, picture menus

Directions   1. Follow these simple directions:

- Look at these alphabet cards. Give me the letter that comes after **B** and the letter that comes after **N**.
- Turn over the alphabet cards that come before **Z** and before **B**.
- Put your finger on the first word in the second paragraph of the third chapter in this book.
- Tell me the letters and the sounds of those letters in your name.

2. Here are some pictures of food you might order in a restaurant. The price of each item is given below the picture. Look at the picture menu and tell me what you would order and what it would cost. Now turn the picture menu over and repeat your order and the prices.

3. Listen carefully to these riddles. When I am through I want you to repeat them to me–then I will tell you the answers if you don't know them.

- How many letters are in the alphabet?   (24–L & M got kicked out for smoking)
- How did the octopus go into battle?   (well armed)
- What is worse than finding a worm in an apple? (finding half a worm)

4. Repeat these rhymes after me:

- I think it is fun to jump and run.
- In one sandwich I have ham; in the other I have jam.

Evaluation:

Task	Number correct	Kinds of errors
1		
2		
3		
4		

Variations: Obtain more varied menus. Have the child select his or her own riddle book from the library and rehearse more difficult riddles. Memorize poems and rhymes.

Objective: to recall initial and final consonant sounds and use them in sentences

Materials: lowercase picture-consonant cards, tape recorder

Directions: Look at these ten picture-alphabet cards that are arranged in a mixed-up order on the chalkboard:

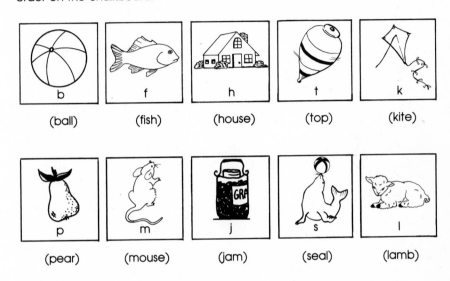

| b | f | h | t | k |
| (ball) | (fish) | (house) | (top) | (kite) |

| p | m | j | s | l |
| (pear) | (mouse) | (jam) | (seal) | (lamb) |

1. Turn on the tape recorder. Pick an alphabet card and tell me in order:
   - the name of the letter.
   - the sound of the letter in picture presented.
   - the name of the picture.
   - the sound of the letter and **another** word where you also hear the sound in the same place.

2. Now turn the cards over and hand me one at a time. I will look and tell you the letter name and then you tell me the sound, the picture word, and the other word you mentioned earlier.

3. Pick a letter card. Tell me a word using that letter sound and then use it in a sentence.

continued

4. Look at the letter picture cards below:

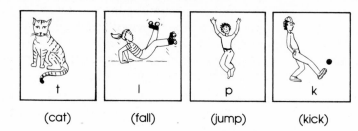

<table>
<tr><td>t</td><td>l</td><td>p</td><td>k</td></tr>
<tr><td>(cat)</td><td>(fall)</td><td>(jump)</td><td>(kick)</td></tr>
</table>

Now tell me the name of the letter, the picture word, and how the letter sounds at the **end** of the word. Now I will tell you one of these letters. Use it as the final sound in a word at the end of a sentence.

Evaluation:

Task	Number correct	Kinds of errors
1		
2		
3		
4		

Variations: Use letters **r, v, d, g, c, n, w, z, x, q.** Have the child play back the tape and correct errors. Record other words and sentences with specified sounds.

Heilman (1964) confirms that a phonics teaching program should be part of all good reading instruction but warns that phonics is but one part of the total word-analysis program and that children can be taught overreliance on sounding out words, which is an inefficient procedure by itself. Beginning reading instruction should foster the idea that reading is a meaning-making process and must include visual integration, structural analysis, and contextual learning.

The special importance of emphasizing meaning in auditory-vocal synthesis instruction for reading-disabled children is discussed by Wallach and Goldsmith (1977), who advocate a three-step approach as follows:

1. using sentence structure and syntax in synthesizing smaller units and then reading for meaning

2. teaching words in context

3. teaching syllabic sound units, meaningful segments, and information units for generalization and abstractions (for example: "walked" means "walk plus past tense")

It has been particularly difficult to teach auditory-vocal synthesis skills to dyslexic children. This process is essentially one of language development which is prerequisite to formal reading. Wiig and Semel (1976, p. 77) give an excellent review of programs and techniques for remediating perceptual-linguistic processing deficiencies. They specify a number of critical segmentation and syllabication skills commonly requiring remediation:

- forming words out of different phonemes

- predicting and formulating words when phonemes or syllables are missing

- identifying separate words that are parts of component words

- identifying the number of syllables in words of different length

- identifying the position of stressed syllables in multisyllabic words

- identifying initial and final syllables of multisyllabic words

- identifying stressed and unstressed syllables

These aural language skills should be developed in dyslexic children before they are taught regular reading. Intensive sequential lessons with adequate opportunity for feedback and self-correction should be a part of the remedial strategy. Other relevant language skills (such as the learning of prefixes, suffixes, and basic semantics) have also been outlined in some detail by Wiig and Semel (1976).

Of course, numerous phonic instructional systems have been devised to teach the more fundamental auditory-vocal synthesis skills required in reading. Several of these have been created for persons with severe reading disorders and are unique in their structure and intensity. Serio and Briggs (1967–68) devised an auditory approach to phonics instruction (for use with minimally neurologically handicapped children in experimental classes) that begins with simple sound discrimination, moves to the isolation of syllables in nonsense words, and finally makes transition to listening activities in meaningful words and sentences. Seventeen sequential steps and lessons are presented for developing vowel auditory discrimination, unvoiced consonant auditory discrimination, and voiced consonant auditory discrimination. Similarly, Price and Price (1977), at the Portland Training College for the Disabled near Nottingham, England, created a fifteen-stage, twenty-six-week phonics program (including forty-one tapes and fifteen workbooks) that was highly successful with more than four hundred "hopelessly illiterate adults." Trela (1968) summarizes a number of different remedial techniques that include special lessons using phonics, tape recorders, and other auditory-vocal synthesis techniques.

Traub and Bloom (1972) outline a highly systematic phonics approach found to be very useful in treating severe reading disabilities. Their program is an adaptation of the Orton-Gillingham method, which is discussed in Chapter 9. The Traub and Bloom program consists of a series of developmental "recipes" in sequential lesson form that begin with consonants and then proceed through consonant blends, syllables, vowels, and affixes. A good summary of the critical word-analysis skills that should be sequentially taught in all intensive remedial reading programs is given by Roswell and Natchez (1977, p. 121):

1. sight words (Dolch)

2. initial consonants: *s, d, m, t, h, p, f, c, r, b, l, n, g, w, j, k, v, y, z*

3. short vowel sounds: *a, i, o, u, e*

4. consonant digraphs: *sh, ch, th*

5. consonant blends: *sm, sp, st, tr, gr, br, cl, fl*

6. long vowel sounds; the silent *e*; and vowel digraphs

7. syllabication

Some of the auditory-vocal synthesis programs and instructional materials frequently used in clinical and prescriptive-special education are listed below:

GOAL Language Development Program (Milton Bradley Company) is a systematic language development program created on the ITPA model for use with young children. It includes special lessons in sound blending, auditory closure, grammatic closure, auditory reception, auditory association, and auditory sequential memory. In this program the auditory-vocal synthesis skills are programmed as an integral part of other language processing abilities.

Recipe for Reading (Educators Publishing Service), by Traub and Bloom, is a practical guide for remedial specialists attempting to relate auditory-vocal synthesis skills to functional phonics and reading. One of the best manuals of its kind.

Phonics We Use Games (Lyons and Carnahan) is a valuable set of ten games for use with reading-disabled children. Games include:

1. Old Itch (initial consonant sounds)
2. Spin-A-Sound (initial consonant sounds and symbols)
3. Bingobang (final consonant sounds and symbols)
4. Blends Race (initial consonant blends and symbols)
5. Digraph Whirl (initial consonant digraphs and symbols)
6. Digraph Hopscotch (initial and final consonant digraphs and symbols)
7. Vowel Dominoes (long and short vowels and symbols)
8. Spin Hard, Spin Soft (hard and soft sounds of *c* and *g*)
9. Full House (vowels, vowel digraphs, diphthongs)
10. Syllable Count (syllabication and accent)

Structural Reading Series (L. W. Singer Company) has colorful workbooks that help children to develop sound-symbol association and integration in beginning phonics training. It can be used as part of an overall phonics approach advocated by its author Catherine Stern (1976).

Following are examples of exercises in auditory-vocal synthesis.

Objective: to synthesize and recall symbol sequences

Materials: symbol, letter, and picture cards

Directions: 1. **Visual recall of auditory patterns.** Listen carefully to these rhythmic taps (•) and then show me the correct card for each one:

    • •   •   • •

    • • •   • •   •

    •   • •   •   • •   •

2. **Motor reproduction of tapped-out rhythmic patterns.** Close your eyes and listen to these taps on the table–then you tap out the pattern you hear:

    •   • • •   •

    • •   • •   • • •   •

    • • •   • •   •   • • • •

3. **Verbal reproduction of letter patterns.** Close your eyes and listen to the sounds I make. Then repeat them after me:

    b b   b   b b   s   s s   s s s

    c c c   c c   c   d   d d   d   d d   d

    a a   b   a b   t t t   a b   s d

4. **Temporal order of visual letter sequences.** Look closely at these letter cards and remember them as I show them to you one at a time (show each letter and then turn it over):

    1. [A] [C] [B]
    2. [B] [X] [T] [E]
    3. [R] [D] [O] [P] [E]

    Now I will show you a letter and you tell me when–in what order–you saw it (1st, 2nd, 3rd, 4th, 5th).

5. **Temporal order of pictures.** Listen carefully to the words I say. After you hear them I will give you this pack of picture cards. Then you give me the pictures of the words in the order that I said them:

    • 1. dog   2. boat

    • 1. car   2. house   3. snake

    • 1. shoes   2. tree   3. cat   4. bicycle

    • 1. book   2. cake   3. milk   4. elephant   5. airplane

Evaluation: Number and kinds of errors for each task.

Variations: Have students design their own exercises.

Objective: to identify vowel sounds in words

Materials: vowel picture cards

Directions:

1. **Short vowels.** Look at these short vowel picture cards. The sounds in the picture are at the beginning of the words–say the sounds and the word:

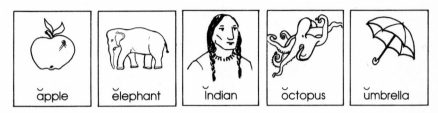

| ăpple | ĕlephant | ĭndian | ŏctopus | ŭmbrella |

Now I am going to say some nonsense words. Listen to the sound in the **middle** of the word–it will be a short vowel sound. Repeat the entire word, then say the vowel sound for me and point to that vowel card. For example, if I say **zap**, the sound is **a** and I point to the card like this. Here are the other words:

kex	belt	cam	kib	pat
dif	box	gud	let	nog
lut	cap	zip	rem	mab
rom	fish	tef	nim	not
zax	jug	cut	kep	lum

| ă | ĕ | ĭ | ŏ | ŭ |

continued

2. **Long vowels:** Look at these colored long vowel cards:

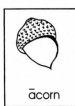

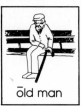
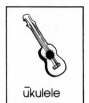

| ācorn | ēagle | īce cream | ōld man | ūkulele |

This time I will say some more nonsense words. Listen again to the sound in the middle of the word–now it will be a long vowel sound. Repeat the word after me, then say the vowel sound by itself and point to that vowel card. Remember that long vowels say their own names:

pie	glode	slote	sprate	cake
fuse	cane	hoe	drupe	stime
stame	slide	plebe	tie	drite
skune	grele	prame	clibe	whale
mice	frume	cage	smode	plene

ā	ē	ī	ō	ū

Evaluation:

	Number correct	Kinds of errors
Long vowels		
Short vowels		

Variations: Use tape-recorded lessons and have children conduct self-evaluations. Have them make their own list of nonsense and real words.

Objective: to be able to hear and locate syllables in words

Materials: worksheet, electric vibrator

Directions: 1. Listen carefully. A syllable may be a single vowel or a group of letters that includes a vowel. A syllable is a unit that can be pronounced. For example, these words are single-syllable words:

car   joy   pig   key   put

This time I will say the one-syllable word and rub your forearm with this vibrator so you can feel the sound as I say it. Now this time you say each word after me and vibrate your arm.

2. Here are two syllable words. Say them after me and vibrate your arm as you say the syllables:

cam' el   doc' tor   mush' room   li' on

mag' net   ham' mer   hel' met

3. Here are three-syllable words. Say them after me and vibrate your arm as you pronounce each syllable:

di' no saur   pro jec' tor   but' ter fly   pi an' o   hand' ker chief

ba nan' a   to ma' to   oc' to pus   val' en tine

4. Now listen carefully as I say a word. Then you say the word **silently to yourself** but rub your arm for each syllable and tell me how many syllables are in the word:

pig   cam' el   di' no saur   skel' e ton   skis

cher' ries   bath' tub   cal' en dar   rose

Evaluation:

Task	Number correct	Kinds of errors
1		
2		
3		
4		

Variations: Use four and five-syllable words. Substitute mechanical hand buzzer for electric vibrator. Break simple sentences into syllables. Systematically teach rules: (a) there are as many syllables in a word as vowel sounds, (b) in case of two adjacent consonants the syllables are divided between them.

SUMMARY   In this chapter we have discussed some of the major auditory processing deficiencies found in dyslexic children including auditory reception, auditory decoding, auditory memory, and auditory-vocal synthesis problems. Ample research proves that specific auditory skills can be developed. Auditory-processing skill deficiencies can also be remediated with systematic prescriptive instruction.

Most of the remedial programs reviewed in this chapter also involve other modalities such as visual and kinesthetic skills. Several sample lessons have been presented that illustrate techniques and procedures used in successful programs. With dyslexic children, the most effective remedial auditory techniques provide intensive learning experience and prompt feedback through multisensory devices and machines.

DISCUSSION QUESTIONS AND ACTIVITIES

1. Discuss the most significant deficiency found in dyslexic children.
2. Define *dysacusis*.
3. Read and discuss one of the research studies summarized by Spache.
4. Use a binaural auditory trainer with a dyslexic child and record the amplification used in each ear over several lessons on different days.
5. Use Rohr's simultaneous procedure with separately taped stories and separate earphones. Which ear was more proficient in decoding the story, answering questions, and so forth?
6. How might "music therapy" be used with dyslexic children?
7. Demonstrate and discuss one of the commercially available programs described in this chapter.
8. What is morphology? Why is it important in the education of dyslexic children?
9. Develop a detailed lesson for teaching a specific auditory processing skill to a learning-handicapped child. Teach the lessons and discuss the skills.
10. Study the auditory subtest of the Slingerland Screening Test. How could this subtest be used as a pretest or posttest for prescriptive teaching?

11. List several books of simple rhymes, poems, and riddles that might be used for auditory memory training of dyslexic children.

12. What is the best predictive reading test to use with primary grade children?

13. Present a detailed review of the Wiig and Semel (1976) approach to remediating auditory processing deficiencies.

14. Why do dyslexic children have so much difficulty with syllabication?

It has proved advisable to make
sure of all of the usable linkages
between vision, audition, and kin-
esthesis while the reading retrain-
ing is under way.

Samuel Orton

CHAPTER NINE

Special
Multisensory Reading Methods

Samuel Orton, a pediatric neurologist, was intimately involved with the
diagnosis and treatment of children with severe reading disorders. As a
result of his extensive clinical work, Orton (1937) advocated a multisensory approach to the remediation of dyslexia. Consequently, although
some programs do stress the development of visual or auditory processing
skills, almost all practical remedial methodologies are multisensory ones.

Experimental studies support the multisensory approach. Many of
these have already been discussed in this book. Fundamental research
in perception, such as that reported by Ittelson and Kilpatrick (1951),
shows that what we perceive and understand is based on relevant and
consistent multisensory experience and action. Spache (1976) reviewed
numerous perceptual studies and concludes that reading is an intersensory process involving many visual, auditory, muscular, and cross modality associations; therefore, multimodal methods should be used in
remedial instruction. Other investigators, such as Hallahan and Cruickshank (1973, p. 174), have reviewed numerous statistical studies and
conclude that visual-perceptual disabilities in the early grades and visual-auditory disabilities in the later grades may be at the root of reading disability and that "empirical evidence warrants the exploration of
multisensory perceptual training for such children."

Since it is impossible to review all multisensory programs and methods in this chapter, only those directly relevant to the remediation of dyslexic children will be considered. These have been grouped into four major categories: simultaneous association (Orton-Gillingham), psychoneurological impress, kinesthetic, and perceptual-motor. Of course these are somewhat artificial divisions since considerable overlap exists in all multisensory approaches.

SIMULTANEOUS ASSOCIATION (ORTON-GILLINGHAM)

Orton's approach to reading was developmental. To him, language was an evolving function developing from a hierarchy of complex integrations in the nervous system and culminating in unilateral control by one (usually the left) of the two brain hemispheres (Orton 1966). Dyslexic children have difficulty in the association process with conflict between the two hemispheres that produces confusion, orientation problems, and a delay in learning to read. Orton noted that reading-disabled children could see, recognize, and even copy some words correctly but failed to identify them as meaningful language symbols and could not associate them with the spoken words. Remedial training in Orton's program is based on tracing and sounding the word-symbol and maintaining consistent ocular sequencing by following the letters with a finger during the sound synthesis of syllables and words.

These remedial principles were translated into an educational method by two of Orton's teacher colleagues, Bessie Stillman and Anna Gillingham. The basis for their remedial lessons was the *simultaneous association* and use of visual, auditory, and kinesthetic language stimuli. Beginning lessons teach individual letters and phonemes, proceed to syllabication and the synthesis of letter-sound patterns, and culminate in phrase and sentence reading. Emphasis is on the combined use of motor elements in speech and writing activities. Through the use of simultaneous techniques, the child learns how a letter or word looks, how it sounds, how the speech organs feel in pronouncing it, and how the hand feels in writing the grapheme or word.

A teacher's manual by Gillingham and Stillman (1965) elaborates on this method and presents a series of highly structured lessons involving the following sequence:

1. The student is shown the printed letter and repeats its name after the teacher.

2. The teacher says the letter sound and the student repeats it.

3. The student watches the teacher write the letter and then traces the teacher's model.

4. The student copies the teacher's model.

5. The student writes the letter or word from memory.

6. The student writes the symbol in the air with eyes closed.

7. The student writes the symbol in normal size on regular paper.

8. The teacher says the letter name and the student responds with the sound of the letter.

Several variations have been made on the Orton-Gillingham method by other special educators. Stuart (1963) reports extensive research findings supporting this method. Stuart stresses the neurophysiological benefits of supplementing the Orton-Gillingham method with body orientation and memory games together with speech practice in matching, classifying, and reproducing stories. In a study of various treatment approaches to dyslexia, Johnson (1969) advocates the use of intrasensory compensatory techniques for visual and auditory dyslexia: visual dyslexics profited from color cues, increased letter size, verbalization, and tactile guides; auditory dyslexics gained most from rhyming-blending-sequencing tasks *with eyes closed,* learning sight words, binaural amplifiers, and the combined use of kinesthetic approaches. Tarnopol and Tarnopol (1976) report that the Orton-Gillingham method is among the most frequently used in remedial programs throughout the world although it stresses alphabetic phonics rather than whole word "gestalt" methods.

A major study involving this method was conducted by Wilson, Harris, and Harris (1976). This program involved 380 elementary school students from twenty-one schools divided into four experimental groups. The students were diagnosed as having significant auditory perceptual deficiencies according to the Lindamood Auditory Conceptualization Test. A number of different remedial programs were used including the Gillingham, Auditory Discrimination in Depth (ADD), Sullivan Programmed Reading, and some combinations of these. Posttest scores on the Woodcock Reading Mastery Tests for Word Identification and Word Attack showed that the Gillingham method produced gains in reading. However, even more effective results were achieved when this method was combined with the ADD program.

An extensive modification of this method was made by Beth Slingerland (1967), who introduced developmental games and exercises including speech, auditory recall, visual recall, kinesthetic recall, and left-right orientation lessons for use with young children. Slingerland (1969) also devised a series of developmental criterion tests for use with this program as follows:

Test 1. chart copying (far point)

Test 2. page copying (near point)

Test 3. visual perceptual memory (marking symbols on a page from memory)

Test 4. visual discrimination (direct symbol matching)

Test 5. visual perceptual kinesthetic memory (reproducing designs from memory)

Test 6. auditory recall (writing numbers, letters, words from dictations)

Test 7. auditory sound discrimination (writing sounds at the beginning and end of words)

Test 8. auditory visual association (selecting words from a dictated list)

Test 9. repeating words and phrases and "cloze" sentences (contextual memory and understanding)

The Slingerland approach is published in a teacher's guide (Slingerland 1971). It emphasizes multisensory learning of advanced symbolic material including oral reading of phrases and sentences and listening to recorded stories while simultaneously reading them aloud. Other modifications of this method have been made by diagnostic-prescriptive specialists such as Porterfield (1976). Another educator, Englemann (1969), has programmed the steps required to translate written symbols into appropriate sounds and has produced the DISTAR program, which contains workbooks and very highly structured multisensory lessons.

The major instructional materials available for teaching the Orton-Gillingham method are available from Educators Publishing Service, Inc. and include the following items:

Remedial Training for Children with Specific Disability in Reading, Spelling, and Penmanship, second edition, a manual by Anna Gillingham and Bessie Stillman, contains lessons introducing letters and building letter sounds into words. Accompanying materials include phonics drill cards, phonetic word cards, syllable cards, diphthong cards, little story books, and a special dictionary set.

A Multisensory Approach to Language Arts for Specific Language Disability Children—A Guide for Primary Teachers and **Basics in Scope and Sequence: A Guide for Primary Teachers in the Second-Year Continuum,** two volumes by Beth Slingerland, are supplemented by alphabet wall cards, patterns for tracing letters of the alphabet, small manuscript alphabet cards, and a teacher's word list.

Following is one example of an exercise in simultaneous association.

PSYCHONEUROLOGICAL IMPRESS METHODS

Several multisensory methods have been devised that attempt to overcome faulty habit patterns detrimental to proficient learning. For example, many dyslexic children do not pay attention to what they read, quickly lose their place, and then make erratic oral responses. Intensive drills may be used to "break through" old behavior patterns and to make new impressions on the central nervous system. These techniques are usually referred to as "impress" methods.

One of the early experiments with this method was conducted by Heckelman (1969) and his colleagues, who reported highly significant gains for students on the Gray Oral Reading Test. Heckelman refers to his approach as the Neurological Impress Method (N.I.M.). It requires fifteen minutes a day of special instruction for a total of between eight and twelve hours. The procedure follows:

- For a new student, select a reading book approximately one grade level below actual achievement.

- The instructor sits slightly behind the student and to the side, and then begins to read sentences from the book aloud, underlining each word with a finger as it is pronounced.

- The instructor then rereads the material as the student follows. The student now points to the words being read (instructor may hold and direct the child's hand).

- Sentences, phrases, and paragraphs are then repeated until a normal, fluid reading pattern is established.

With this method emphasis is on fluidity and patterning of oral response. No attempt is made to teach sounds of letters or words or to

Objective: to identify, say, write, and use the **s** sound meaningfully

Materials: worksheet, letter card, chalkboard

Directions: 1. Teacher: Here is a card with a letter on it:

It is the letter **s**. Now you tell me its name.

Pupil's Response:

2. Teacher: The letter **s** sound is the snake sound like this: "sss." Now you tell me the sound.

Pupil's Response:

3. Teacher: Watch me write the letter **s** on the chalkboard. Now I will write it in this box:

Now you **trace** my **s** on the chalkboard and box.

4. Copy the letter **s** several times on the line below:

5. Now I will cover the letter **s** so you cannot see it. Write the letter **s** several times on the line below:

6. Close your eyes. Write the letter **s** in the air in front of your face. Now do it again keeping your eyes closed and saying the sound of the letter **s**.

7. Here is your regular lined paper. Write the letter **s** on the line several times and say the sound as you do so.

8. What is the sound that the letter **s** makes? Tell me some words that begin with the letter **s** sound.

Evaluation: Circle correct steps made. Kinds of errors:

Variations: Have the student use salt or sand trays or fingerpaint for kinesthetic feedback. Use a tape recorder and play back response. Introduce other letters and sounds.

correct the student. As the student develops confidence and rhythmic response, other reading material such as newspaper stories, magazines, and self-selected, high-interest books should be introduced. Heckelman (1976) states that if reading improvement is not noted within four hours, this method should be supplemented with kinesthetic and other techniques. This approach appears to be helpful with reading-disabled children because it exposes them to many words in a patterned context. An ordinary fifteen minute session should cover up to two thousand words or ten to twenty pages of reading material.

With dyslexic children, use tape recorders and other equipment to enrich this method. The instructor might read into the child's right ear while the child speaks into a microphone. The child's voice is amplified for immediate feedback and recorded for later playback and evaluation. A variation is to combine this approach with the stereo-reader apparatus, which increases visual impress and improves lateral dominance. Later, children can use their own acquired vocabulary to write (or dictate) stories, which they then reread using neuropsychological impress methods.

These methods have also been used with older students. Van den Honert (1977) reports one such program involving neuropsychological techniques with dyslexics in junior high school. Her program was a unique combination of methods that included:

- a systematic phonics program emphasizing syllabication and using manipulatives such as letter-sound tiles, phonic cards, and similar materials
- visual training of symbols and words using specially occluded glasses to help imprint perceptions in the left hemisphere
- binaural earphones with the left ear (right hemisphere) receiving music and the right ear (left hemisphere) simultaneously receiving taped reading and spelling material
- right-hand tactile spelling of words on raised kinesthetic tiles placed under the desk (and out of sight)

As a result of these techniques, Van den Honert was able to impress symbolic-linguistic material on the left hemisphere of her experimental students, who showed a four-year gain on the Gilmore Oral Reading Test scores (the gain was two and a half times that of the control group). Although it is easy to criticize the design and techniques of Van den Honert's experiment, the study illustrates the many possible approaches to using neuropsychological impress methods.

Luria (1963) also conducted experimental rehabilitation programs with reading-disabled persons who had brain injuries. He advocates the use of multisensory approaches that might help to impress visual and auditory patterns of letters and words and thereby improve gestalt organization in the brain. Through exercises and reeducation tasks, such as sequential rhythmic-reading patterns, brain function is reorganized and cognition is restored.

There are no ready-made commercial programs or kits containing psychoneurological impress methods. This method must be adapted by the instructor to the specific needs of the student using any suitable equipment, books, and materials. There are, though, several kinds of machines that can be used as learning aids to help impress visual-auditory patterns on the central nervous system. Some of these are listed below:

Keystone Integrator (Keystone View Company) is a simple but useful machine that requires the child to look at visual targets, such as pictures, designs, numbers, letters, or phonic signs and then to activate a flashing light and audio-tone pattern by pressing four switches with both hands and both feet. Correct responses produce a smooth pleasing tone and light pattern. Incorrect responses result in a harsh tone (negative reinforcement). This apparatus can also be used with a tape recorder to provide audio feedback of oral reading material.

Video Arcade Games (Sears Stores) are among the several new video games requiring visual-motor-audio coordination and integration. These games are attached to television sets or obtained in special cartridge-cassette game forms and provide moving targets, sounds, running scores, and symbolic information. The games may be used with sports stories or students' own stories to help impress multisensory patterns.

Franzblau Multisensory Coordinator (Keystone View Company) is a visual training machine that has light-sensing pens with which students trace designs, letters, and words on an illuminated screen. When the pen is off-target a light goes off, a tone is sounded, and an electric counter records the error made. Several special "game" programs, which include Dolch basic vocabulary words, advanced word groups, and other lessons, are available for use with this machine.

An example of an exercise using the neurological impress method follows.

Objective: to be able to experience, through multisensory stimulation, normal rhythmic sound patterns while reading common sentences

Materials: sentence strips, word cards, tape recorder

Directions:

1. Look at the sentence strips that I will show you one at a time. Point quietly to each word in the strip.

2. Now listen carefully while I read the sentence in your right ear and then watch how I point to each word as I say it.

3. Turn on the tape recorder. Now we will say the sentences together. I will say them just a little bit faster than you do. Point to each word as you read it:

   a. Valentine's day is in February.

   b. On the Fourth of July we go on a picnic to the park.

   c. Halloween is in October and we like to go out at night for "tricks or treats."

   d. On Thanksgiving day in November, we usually have turkey and pumpkin pie to eat.

   e. When Christmas day comes in December, I am always in a hurry to open my presents.

4. Now listen to the playback on the tape recorder. Point to each word again as you hear it.

5. Use these word cards and arrange the words to match each of the sentences we have read. This time we will read them again but faster. Point to the words as you read them.

6. This time read each sentence by yourself. Point to each word as you read it. Now listen to yourself on the tape.

Evaluation: Record time and kinds of errors made.

Variations: Use basal reading books. Underline words using penlight. Have the child write sentences.

KINESTHETIC METHODS

Some children learn best when they are able to touch, feel, and kinesthetically experience the sounds or words presented to them. Kinesthetic methods provide immediate feedback and permit quick correction of errors. Jastak and Jastak (1976, p. 90) state that if dyslexic children are allowed to trace letters, move lips, or engage in motor responses using both sides of the body, there occurs a reporting back to the unilateral language center. They believe that "the ease of overcoming reading difficulties depends on how early feedback channels are developed."

A systematic kinesthetic method for teaching reading-disabled children was developed a number of years ago by Grace Fernald (1943) at the University of California, Los Angeles, Psychological Clinic school. Fernald concludes that "a large percentage of cases" of extreme reading disability come about because of teaching that omits kinesthetic cues, for example, the deliberate suppression of motor adjustments, such as lip, throat, and hand movements in reading. Dyslexic children were found to exhibit negative emotional attitudes to reading and displayed deficiencies in visual-auditory perception, failure in discriminating phonemes, and associated confusions in reading and writing (such as inverting or reversing letters and words). Through the use of structured kinesthetic methods almost all reading-disabled children were able to make highly significant gains. The steps in this method are outlined below:

1. On a single sheet of paper the instructor writes the word to be learned in two-inch letters.

2. The instructor tells the student the word and pronounces each syllable.

3. The student traces the word with a finger and at the same time sounds it out.

4. The student copies the word and pronounces it.

5. The student writes the word from memory and pronounces it.

Each of the above steps is repeated until the child masters the word. No erasures are permitted since the emphasis is on learning the whole word as a gestalt unit. (That is also why cursive writing is most often used with the method.) Later the child keeps a word file, makes up stories, and then has them typed out for future use.

Fernald supplemented the method with other multisensory techniques such as the use of shallow, colored baking pans or boxes containing salt or sand for finger writing. Most special educators use adaptations of this method in prescriptive education. One of the most interesting reports on the success of the method was made by Seagoe (1965), who details a clinical study of a mongoloid boy who began Fernald kinesthetic reading training when he was seven years old and finally reached a seventh-grade performance level when he was forty-three years old. (He was also able to write regularly to friends.)

Some other kinesthetic approaches have been devised for use with dyslexic children. In a report on successful prescriptive programs, Blanco (1972) recommends the usual structured multisensory-phonetic program but also advocates that the extreme dyslexic be taught using special equipment and even Braille materials. McCoy (1975) used Braille with a severely dyslexic fifteen-year-old girl of normal vision. Braille lessons were held one hour a day for seven months, and her significant improvement was attributed to kinesthetic input that improved central processing skills and cognition.

In his book on dyslexia, Jordan (1972) states that of the types of dyslexia, visual dyslexia is most prevalent and auditory dyslexia most difficult to correct. He recommends structured lessons and sequential learning exercises that help imprint sound-symbol associations and advocates that the child typewrite five words, read them into a tape recorder, and then replay them.

A study done by Campbell (1973) hypothesizes that typewriting substituted for handwriting would reduce "proprioceptive errors and interference" common to learning-disabled children and thereby improve academic performance. He compared forty experimental children in five special education classes with forty control children in special classes. The same reading materials and instructions were given to both groups over a three-month period. But children in the experimental group were introduced to "hunt and peck" typing and did not use pencils at any time for any activity at school during the treatment period. Reading vocabulary score gains on the Gates-MacGinitie Reading Tests in the experimental group were double those in the control group although no significant gains were made in reading comprehension. Recommendations were made to (a) teach such children visual discrimination skills by typing letters, (b) have the children type words and simple stories and copy them in manuscript form, and (c) then engage the children in cursive writing of learned words and sentences.

In another related program, Slayback (1975) found that although her learning-disabled students gained in phonics and word-recognition skills from prescriptive instruction, they lacked interest in reading and real understanding of what they had read. Slayback had her students write books based on their personal experiences and paid them for doing so. The books were bound and then read by their authors to their parents and to children in younger classes. General reading achievement improved significantly as did other language arts activities. Inattentive behaviors also decreased. Apparently the kinesthetic act of writing with immediate reinforcement and multisensory stimulation resulted in more meaningful organization and integration of material being read.

Similarly, Connell (1977) studied nineteen experimental kindergarten classes where children were taught to write lowercase letters as they were introduced. Sensory-motor activities accompanied all writing tasks. Compared with children in twenty-six control classes, the experimental groups did significantly better on end-of-year word and sentence reading tests. The program was then used with multihandicapped children and achieved equal success.

There can be no doubt that kinesthetic techniques such as letter and word tracing, copying, typing, writing, and recording all provide direct practice in reading. The multisensory feelings provided by finger touching and small muscle feedback combined with visual and auditory discrimination tasks give direction to the learning process in dyslexic children. Again, most kinesthetic teaching materials are largely teacher-made or adaptations of instructional aids such as those listed below.

Kinesthetic Alphabet (R. H. Stone Products) is a set of upper and lowercase white-sand letters mounted on a black cardboard backing. These and other kinesthetic letters (plastic, wooden, felt, magnetic, and others) are available in all teacher supply houses and should be a part of all special educators' resource materials.

STEP Language Board and Language Strips (L. A. Hatch Company) is a multisensory approach to decoding and encoding words that uses a plastic board with colored interlocking language word strips. Sequential lessons teach letters representing beginning, ending, and medial sounds and provide some practice in beginning spelling. Handwriting is introduced through tracing experiences.

Reading via Typing (AVKO) is a series of unique typing lessons for learning-disabled students. The lessons use "word family phonics" to help students improve their reading and spelling skills. Other audio, visual, kinesthetic, and oral (AVKO) instructional materials are also available for use with this program.

An example of a kinesthetic exercise follows.

PERCEPTUAL-MOTOR METHODS

One of the earliest successful perceptual-motor training programs was devised by Jean Itard (1894/1962). Itard conducted prescriptive instruction with a ten-year-old "wild boy" named Victor who completely lacked human language. Beginning with multisensory activities designed to develop Victor's senses of sight and touch, Itard trained the boy to read and write a series of sight words and then to decode and analyze what he was reading. The initial teaching method stressed distinguishing objects and letters by touch and developing comprehension and meaning through direct life applications. Since Itard's time many other perceptual-motor reading programs have been devised and tried.

In a symposium on the identification and treatment of learning disorders in school children, Krippner (1965) reported on a remedial study of poor readers with central nervous system perceptual dysfunctions. Forty-eight children from seven years, eleven months through seventeen years, three months old were enrolled in a five-week summer remedial clinic. A total perceptual-motor program included the use of self-reinforcement techniques, sandpaper letters, touch boards, magnetic slates, consonant and vowel flash cards, word wheels, basic word lists, experience stories, programmed materials, high-interest literature, and book writing. In addition, special lessons were introduced using visual tracking materials, eye-hand coordination tasks, and stereo-reader training. Prescriptive activities used with children included map making, desensitization, educational hypnosis, and bibliotherapy. The mean improvement for the group on the California Reading Test was 5.64 months, and one student made almost a two-year gain.

A detailed clinical report by Early and Kephart (1969) on a ten-year-old boy enrolled in the reading clinic of the Achievement Center for Children at Purdue University helps to illustrate other successful

Objective: to type and read back simple sentences and stories

Materials: primary typewriter, tape recorder, and earphones

Directions:

1. Here is a typewriter with a sheet of paper in it with your name typed on it. Here is the key with the first letter of your name which is _____. I will type it on this paper. Now you say the letter and type a line.

2. Now I will tell and show you the other letters in your name and where to find the type keys. Then you type a line of letters for each one I show you.

3. Watch while I put all of the letters together and type your name. Now you type your name several times on the next line.

4. On this new sheet of paper I will type "Christmas is in December." Now point to each word as we read the sentence together. Do it again. Look carefully at the word **Christmas** and tell me each letter. As you tell me the letter I will show you where to find it on the keyboard so you can type each letter and word in the sentence.

5. Read to me the sentence that you have just typed. Point to each word as you read it.

6. Now put this earphone on your right ear and turn on the tape recorder. You will hear letters you have already typed. When you hear a letter type it ten times.

7. Now tell me a sentence of your own you would like to type. We will retype your sentences on file cards and use them in stories later.

Evaluation: Kinds of errors:

Variations: Have students type Dolch words in short sentences and stories. Illustrate typed stories with drawings and magazine pictures.

perceptual-motor methodologies. Following intensive initial diagnostic-prescriptive evaluation, this boy received nine weeks (forty-five hours) of remediation at the clinic together with home training lessons. Because it was decided that the boy's reading problems stemmed from his lack of neuropsychological organization, he was trained in relaxation, body directional control and orientation, rhythmic coordination, visual pursuit and convergence, following words with fingers, chalkboard exercises, and Fernald-kinesthetic techniques including cursive writing. He made a significant gain in perceptual-motor skills and reading scores. On the Durrell Analysis of Reading Difficulty subtests he showed a gain of more than a year in oral and silent reading, a two-year gain in listening comprehension, and a four-year gain in visual memory for words and phonic spelling.

A similar study was done by McCormick and Poetker (1968) using forty-two underachieving first graders assigned to matched groups. The experimental perceptual-motor group received training twice a week (forty-five-minute periods) for seven weeks. Lessons stressed listening and attention tasks, following directions, verbalization, visualization, and balancing and jumping activities. The experimental group made significant gains over the control group on the Lee-Clark Reading Readiness Test. In a related study, McCormick, Schnobrich, and Footlik (1969) compared an experimental group of thirty-two first graders with thirty-one controls. Experimental training took place in groups of five children for an hour a day, two days a week for nine weeks. Patterned perceptual training activities were used based on Luria's procedures for developing focused attention and self-direction. The children wore blindfolds to increase their attention to proprioceptive and vestibular cues. No significant gains on the Metropolitan Reading Test scores were made by the experimental group as a whole, but children who were reading below grade-level expectancy improved significantly (at the .01 level) in reading compared to the controls.

Other researchers have reached similar conclusions. One investigation by Halliwell and Solan (1972) studied 105 first graders with potential reading problems. The experimental perceptual-motor groups received lessons in tachistoscopic exposure, auditory discrimination, visual-motor chalkboard activities, visual tracking, and other relevant perceptual tasks as well as regular reading instruction. The training period lasted for seven months with twice-a-week sessions of forty-five minutes each. The experimental group gained significantly on the reading comprehension subtest of the Metropolitan Achievement Test. In this study, developmentally and perceptually immature boys made the greatest gains. The results support the use of this multi-sensory approach with young males.

Some multisensory perceptual-motor training lessons and materials of value in developmental and remedial reading are listed below.

Active Learning—Games to Enhance Academic Abilities (Prentice-Hall Media) is a teacher's manual by Bryant Cratty containing games for developing prereading and reading skills. Separate chapters present games for learning auditory and visual skills, letters, letter sounds and spelling, sight word reading, reading sentences, writing, and reading directions.

Developmental Learning Materials (DLM) produces a number of useful perceptual-motor training materials of value in a developmental or remedial reading program. Some of these are:

- visual matching, memory, and sequencing exercises
- letter constancy cards
- noun, verb, rhyming word puzzles
- compound word games
- beginning sound word hunt puzzles

In addition, various word and sentence card games requiring movement and motor skills are available. Most of these materials help integrate the various perceptual stimuli involved in the reading process.

The Valett Perceptual-Motor Transitions to Reading Program (Academic Therapy Publications) is a program of twenty-six highly structured perceptual-motor lessons for learning letter sounds. Each lesson contains twenty multisensory sequential learning tasks that emphasize action word associations for letter sounds and require self-correction. A set of cards and a 128-page workbook structure this program. Letters are introduced in a purposeful order. In addition to learning letter sounds, children are taught to write the letters and to combine them into words. By completing the program students learn the short vowel sounds, all of the initial consonant sounds, and most of the final consonant sounds. They will also have combined them to write more than sixty different words. An example of an exercise from this program follows.

Objective: to learn the initial **m** sound, to use it in speech and reading, and to be able to write the letter

Materials: picture card and worksheet

Directions:

☐ 1. Look at the picture card with the rough letter **m** on it. Watch how I trace the letter **m** with a finger. Now, you trace the letter **m** with your finger three times. Then, check the box.

☐ 2. Look at this letter: its name is **m**. Say **m** and check the box.

☐ 3. Look at this picture. The letter **m** is used at the beginning of the word **move**. Say "move" and check the box.

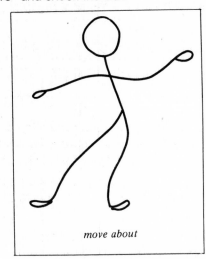

move about

☐ 4. The words and picture say to "move about." Do as it says and check the box.

continued

☐ 5. Listen to me as I say the **sound** of the letter **m**. Now, you say the sound of **m** and check the box.

☐ 6. Color the picture that says "move about" next to number 3, on page 178. Check the box.

☐ 7. Make up your own sentence using the word **move**. Say your sentence out loud and check the box.

☐ 8. Use your **finger** to trace over this letter six times. The arrows will show you which direction to go. As you trace the letter, first say its **name** and then its **sound**, as in **move**. Check the box.

m m m m m m

☐ 9. Now, use your pencil to trace over the above letters. Say the **sound** of the letter as you trace it. Check the box.

☐ 10. Copy the letter **m** five times in the spaces provided. Say the letter's **sound** as you copy it. Check the box.

m				

☐ 11. Now, move about, while you say the **m** sound five times. Check the box.

☐ 12. Write the letter **m** five times from memory. **Don't** look at the one you just finished writing. Say the sound as you write **m**. Check the box.

☐ 13. Trace the word **mat** below. Say the sound of each letter as you trace it.

mat   mat   mat

A door **mat** is something you walk on to clean your feet. Pretend to wipe your feet on a door mat; then check the box.

continued

☐ 14. Draw a picture in the space provided, of some other word that begins with the **m** sound. When you finish, check the box.

[ ]

☐ 15. Tell me three more words that begin with the **m** sound. Check the box when you have given three more words.

☐ 16. Close your eyes. Listen to me read these words. Clap your hands when you hear one that begins with the **m** sound.

| move | kick | man | mouse | turn |
| push | mat | hit | bounce | mischief |

If you clapped your hands at all the **m** sounds, check the box.

☐ 17. Pretend to move like a monster. As you pretend, say the **m** sound five times. Check the box.

☐ 18. Use a crayon to color this letter. Now use some finger paint and make a big letter **m**. Check the box.

[m]

☐ 19. Trace the rough letter **m** on the picture card with your finger three times, while you say the **sound.** Check the box.

____ 20. Count the number of check marks you earned, and write it on the line.

Evaluation: Note specific kinds of errors made.

Variations: **Supplemental lesson**–after letter **m** introduced: Help the student put these letter sounds together to make words. Figure out the words, trace them and then write them and say them two times.

map

him

ham

SUMMARY

A major difficulty for dyslexic children is making meaningful sound-symbol discriminations and associations. They also have trouble in retaining and recalling these associations once they have learned them. Multisensory methods provide varied means of stimulation and feedback that reinforce, strengthen, and integrate basic visual and auditory processing skills.

To help children to learn to read, multisensory programs must teach sound-symbol or perceptual-linguistic associations and their meanings. Simultaneous association, neuropsychological impress, kinesthetic, and perceptual-motor transition methods give the educator a number of techniques for strengthening the grapheme-phoneme association.

It is widely agreed that dyslexic children can be taught much more than simple sight words. The emphasis should be on teaching phonic skills through the use of multisensory techniques, which provide active practice in both word-sound analysis and synthesis. Authorities such as Critchley (1970) advocate the use of discrimination exercises using games and toys that incorporate letters and words, which can in turn be related to interesting and exciting stories and reading material. Many teachers and clinicians have created multisensory programs of proven effectiveness in helping children learn to read. In all effective programs of this type there is a deliberate attempt to develop basic processing skills using eclectic methods and approaches, such as those described here and by Frostig (1968) and other specialists.

However, as Chall (1967) discovered from her study of how children learn to read, the evidence does not endorse any one decoding method or program over another. Studies fail to show that Orton-Gillingham, i.t.a., linguistic approaches, or any single perceptual-motor program is superior to another. Although it is essential for children to know the names and sounds of the letters before beginning formal reading, Chall recommends a phonic code emphasis only as an introduction to reading. But it must be remembered that multisensory methods can best be used to teach essential introductory decoding skills to dyslexic children at this early stage of learning to read.

An approach to teaching initial reading skills through the use of multisensory techniques is presented below:

1. Talk with the children about their interests and experiences. Make a list of words they would like to learn (for example, dog, fight, ghost, football, mother, dance).

2. Write each word in large cursive across regular 8½-by-11 paper.

3. Show the cursive word to the children and pronounce it while tracing it with your finger.

4. Have the children pronounce the word while tracing it with a finger three times.

5. Have the children use the word in a short sentence ("I like ghost stories." "Football is my favorite game.").

6. Have the children act out the word through body movement. If necessary, have them imitate the teacher or another child. Encourage creative body expression.

7. Have the children *trace* over the large cursive word and say the names of the letters as they trace them three times with a pencil, three times with a felt pen, and three times with a crayon.

8. Have the children *copy* the large cursive word three times each with pencil, pen, and crayon, first saying the word and then the letters as they trace them.

9. Using a 3-by-5 file card have the children write the word in large cursive across the middle, saying the word and letters as they write.

10. On the reverse side of the file card have the children draw a picture or cut out and paste on a picture representing the word ("football").

11. Under the picture have the children write the word in small cursive.

12. Ask the children to tell a brief story about the picture word and to share it with a friend. Have children file the card alphabetically in a personal word file box.

13. Using regular lined paper have children write the word three times from memory using as felt pen or crayon.

14. Teach the children to divide the word into syllables. Have them write the word three times on lined paper saying the syllables as they write.

15. Have the children select one of the following multisensory ways of writing the word: chalkboard, fingerpaint, clay tray, tempera paint, salt or sand tray, wood burning, or Elmer's glue. Using a cassette tape recorder, students should:
    a. Say the entire word and write it ("football")
    b. Say the syllables and write the word ("foot-ball")
    c. Say the letter names and write the word ("f-o-o-t-b-a-l-l")

    d. Repronounce the word and write it in the chosen medium once more.

16. Have the children play back their recordings of the word and write the word on regular lined paper as they hear themselves.

17. After they make several word picture cards, have the children combine some of the words into a story. Record the story; if possible have the children write out the story or have the teacher, aide, or parent type it out for future reference in a "personal storybook" that can be used as a source for future words.

18. Have the children write the word in cursive three times and then print it three times. Have them use wooden or other tactile letters to spell out the word.

19. Teach basic phonics: initial consonants, medial consonants, final consonants, blends, vowels. Analyze word errors made by the child and remediate using proper phonetic sound associations.

20. Introduce the structured reading program and basal reading series and supplement it with language experience units stressing personal-social news stories and events.

Teachers should supplement each step as necessary with additional multisensory activities. Use active games, manipulative material, and high-interest books and recordings. For students with significant reading dysfunctions, use intensive auditory memory, decoding, and other processing programs. It helps to pair students with peers or cross-age tutors and to encourage individual creative approaches in following and using these methods.

DISCUSSION QUESTIONS AND ACTIVITIES

1. Discuss Orton's theory about the cause of dyslexia and its implications for treatment.

2. Conduct several remedial reading lessons using the Orton-Gillingham method and evaluate your results.

3. Administer the Slingerland tests (Form A, B, or C) and write three prescriptive teaching objectives based on test results.

4. Discuss the theory behind Heckelman's (1969) neurological impress method.

5. Repeat Van den Honert's lesson with binaural earphones and discuss the results.

6. Demonstrate the Keystone Integrator using letter or phonic cards.

7. What is the main difference between the Fernald kinesthetic method and the Orton-Gillingham method?

8. How might typing best be used to help remediate dyslexia?

9. Obtain a set of lowercase kinesthetic alphabet cards and demonstrate their use in remedial reading with dyslexic children.

10. Write a report on Itard's *Wild Boy of Aveyron.* Pay special attention to his methods for teaching language and reading skills.

11. Who appears to profit most from multisensory instruction? Why?

12. Describe a good perceptual-motor reading program.

From an external, socially organized attention develops the
child's voluntary attention, which in
this stage is an internal, self-regulating process.

L. S. Vygotsky

CHAPTER TEN

Increasing Attention and Motivation

Dyslexic children have trouble sustaining attention when they read, and their impulsive and distractible behavior contributes to failure and frustration. Eventually a child begins to avoid reading situations, but this response conflicts with demands at school and at home. Many dyslexics develop serious anxiety and stress, resulting in apathy, withdrawal, and lack of self-esteem.

Poor attention, anxiety, and stress compound the problems of learning-disabled children. Many studies confirm that the *primary* learning disability of such children is the inability to focus attention and keep in mind several bits of information until they can be synthesized. Ackerman, Peters, and Dykman (1971) found that the learning-disabled scored lower than controls in tests that measure this ability: the WISC mental Arithmetic and Digit Span subtests. Thus, educators should stress strategies for improving attention and reducing anxiety. This chapter is devoted to such strategies.

ANXIETY REDUCTION

The starting point for increasing attention to learning tasks is to reduce the child's anxiety and reluctance to confront the task. No learning can occur if the child avoids reading or remedial instruction. One must develop the child's self-confidence and belief that he or she will be able to learn to read. With increasing self-confidence and success, anxiety is gradually dissipated.

The major problem then is to tap the child's hidden resources. Puharich (1974) summarizes research showing that all persons possess positive energy that can be self-directed or other-directed for continued growth and development. The major steps in this growth process involve (1) helping the person acquire and assert an objective (that is, "I want to learn to read"), (2) visualizing desired results (such as picturing oneself actually reading interesting books), and (3) using multisensory and highly motivating learning techniques. Puharich discusses how such self-directed use of one's positive energies results in brain actions that induce psychobiological changes in the body and effect changes in behavior.

Useful teaching techniques include relaxation, autosuggestion, hypnosis, meditation, positive visualization, systematic desensitization, and other related procedures. Levine's (1976) study of physiological responses in poor readers disclosed a stress reaction with continued rapid heart rate during task confrontation; further, both attention and cognitive processing improve when stress and anxiety are reduced.

Extensive studies of the positive effects of meditation on academic achievement are discussed by Bloomfield, Cain, Jaffe, and Kory (1975). They report that during meditation cellular activity in the body slows down, reducing the need for oxygen. Increased relaxation permits an increased flow of blood to the muscles and decreases the heart's workload. The reduction in blood chemicals that accompany tension and anxiety results in a sense of ease. Finally, the cells of the brain begin to fire in a more synchronous manner, which fosters integrated functioning between lower and higher brain centers and between the left and right hemispheres. These studies conclude that meditation:

- improves brain wave synchrony
- slows heart rate and improves body reaction to stress
- decreases blood pressure
- decreases anxiety
- improves auditory-perceptual discrimination
- increases memory
- improves grade-point averages

A number of meditation and relaxation training programs have proved successful with learning-handicapped children. Linden (1973) conducted a major study with disadvantaged minority children on the effect of meditation on levels of field independence (ability to screen out distracting environmental stimuli), test anxiety, and reading achievement. Twenty-six third-grade children were given thirty-six meditation training sessions (twenty to twenty-five minutes each) over an eighteen-week period. Meditation exercises progressed through stages of quiet relaxation, body centering, deep breathing, and visualization. An experimental group made significant gains over controls in field independence, attention, and anxiety reduction.

In a similar study, Simpson and Nelson (1974) used breathing control to improve attention and reduce hyperactivity among learning-disabled children in the primary grades. Twelve one-hour training sessions were held over three and a half months. Using feedback and token reinforcers, researchers trained the experimental group to watch and control respiration. The results—improved respiration, attention and vigilance test scores—support the use of this kind of training program with children.

It is not always possible, though, for highly anxious children to succeed in meditation and relaxation training programs without much initial direction and structured guidance. Traditionally, this kind of education has been termed "suggestion training" (hypnosis) or directive guidance: training begins with the student receiving directions from the special educator and proceeds to self-suggestions (or autohypnosis). Extensive research on hypnosis by Barber (1960, 1961) and others shows that these suggestive techniques can produce changed EEG patterns, localized vasoconstriction and vasodilation influencing blood circulation, skinn temperature change, cardiac acceleration and deceleration, and elevation or depression of blood glucose. Other studies, such as those of McCord (1955) and Alexandroff (1972), show that in children hypnosis seems to activate self-regulating mechanisms that gradually filter new learnings and insights into consciousness.

Many experimental programs have been reported showing the positive results of suggestion and hypnosis with learning-handicapped children. The March 8, 1963, *New York Times* ran a story of the San Vincenzo boarding school in Bergamo, Italy, where students listened to tape-recorded sugggestions while resting at their desks. The teachers felt the experiment improved receptivity and performance. Krippner (1966) used hypnosis with children in a summer remedial-reading clinic and found that hypnosis contributed to decreased tension, increased motivation, increased interest in reading, and improved concentration and attention. Krippner also used suggestion to facilitate the revisualization and reauditorization of graphic and spoken symbols. This technique resulted in significant gains by the subjects on the California Reading Test. In another study, Jampolsky (1970) used suggestive-relaxation training plus vibratory, touch, and muscle-memory training (pencil on back, finger tracing in stencil letter grooves) and found that his experimental group completely eliminated number and letter reversals, whereas there were no significant changes in the control group.

More recently, Carter and Synolds (1974) demonstrated the value of suggestive relaxation training in reducing reversals in handwriting. Handwriting improved significantly when children were put into a relaxed state. Schpoont (1973) made a presentation to the American Psychological Association advocating the increased use of hypnosis in schools, especially with learning-disabled and behaviorally disturbed children. A number of suggestive techniques have been adapted and incorporated in other closely related programs. Creative yoga and exercise programs for children and young people were devised by Kiss (1971) and by Carr (1973) and resulted in increased self-control and self-esteem in hyperactive learning-disabled children.

Parents also have been successfully involved in suggestive-relaxation training programs for their children. In one study by Lupin, Braud, Braud, and Duer (1976), an experimental program was conducted with thirteen hyperactive children from four different schools in classes for minimally brain-injured children. These students were involved in twenty-minute home-training lessons over a three-month period. Parents were provided with six commercial tapes on relaxation that included visual imagery, desensitization exercises, and behavior management. Scores on the WISC Digit Span and Object Assembly subtests increased significantly, reflecting reduced anxiety and increased attention.

Many special educators use relaxation exercises to help anxious children learn to reduce tension, focus attention, and increase concentration and achievement. Two examples of relaxation lessons are given here. The second sample lesson elaborates on the five major steps in reducing anxiety through relaxation techniques. These may be used as a basis for supplemental lessons. The teacher should modify the lesson language according to the developmental level and needs of the student or group.

Objective: to relax and visualize suggestions

Materials: tape recorder

Directions: In this mental exercise you will begin to learn to relax, to follow suggestions, and to develop your imagination. Sit quietly in your chair with your hands on your lap and get into a comfortable position with both feet on the floor.

1. Close your eyes and imagine that your eyelids are heavy. Keep your eyes closed and listen carefully to my voice and then follow my instructions.

2. You are beginning to feel very relaxed and comfortable. As you listen to my voice you are becoming even more relaxed and comfortable. Your entire body feels comfortably warm and very good.

3. I am going to count slowly from five to one backwards. With each number you will become more and more relaxed but you will not fall asleep. Five – relaxed, four, three – more relaxed, two – very relaxed, one – deeply relaxed! Your arms, legs, neck, and entire body are now very, very relaxed.

4. Listen carefully, keep your eyes closed, remain deeply relaxed and lift up your first finger on your right hand. Good! Now imagine that you have been outside in the hot sun for a long time without any water to drink. Your throat is getting very dry and you are becoming very thirsty. If you can imagine your throat being dry raise your first finger.

5. Now imagine that you are drinking cool water from a glass. How good it tastes! You can feel it going down your throat. Swallow it and feel it going down and satisfying your thirst. As you imagine drinking cool water raise your first finger.

6. You are even more deeply relaxed now and feeling very, very good. Keep your eyes closed, continue to relax, and imagine what I suggest to you. Imagine yourself in a very comfortable chair. You have a new Walt Disney picture-story book on your desk that is about Donald Duck. It looks like a very good and funny book. You are picking up the book and looking at the first page. It is very colorful and funny and as you see it and read it you begin to smile and laugh. Go ahead now and turn over the other pages and read the rest of this little book to yourself. When you have finished reading, close the book and put your head down in your arms on the desk and relax yourself completely until I call you.

7. Very good. In just a minute I will count to three. With each count you will begin to wake up and become alert. When I get to the count of three you will be fully awake, alert, and feeling fine. You will also be able to remember the Donald Duck story you have just imagined. Ready, one, two, three – very good! You are now awake, alert, and feeling fine.

continued

Evaluation: Note the child's ability to comply with suggestions during each step. Have the child relate his or her imagined story about Donald Duck using a tape recorder. Play back the tape and note the child's responses.

Variations: Tape-record all of the directions using a slow but pleasing voice. Have the child listen to directions using earphones and tape recorder. Extend suggestions to imagining specific stories that the child is acquainted with or currently reading.

Objective: to learn how to relax and release tensions through the use of self-suggestion and imagination

Materials: tape recorder

Directions: Sit down in a comfortable chair with both feet on the floor about a foot or so apart. Just sit comfortably and close your eyes and relax.

1. **Tensing.**   As you begin to relax and let go, you may feel better if you move slightly or even squirm about until you find the most comfortable position. You yourself will be giving and receiving these directions for relaxation, and you will remain open and receptive to them since you know there is nothing to fear. As you let yourself go and follow your self-suggestions you will feel comfortably warm, good, and increasingly relaxed.

   Now with your eyes closed and sitting quietly, begin to make a fist of your right hand. Slowly make it as tight as you can, tighter and tighter! You can now feel the tension go up your right arm all the way to your shoulder. Clench your fist tighter . . . make it as tight as you can. Now let go! Relax your fist and arm. As you let go you can actually feel the tension draining away from your hand and arm and it is a good feeling.

   Now clench your left hand and make it as tight as you can. Tighten up your entire left arm. Feel how tight it is becoming, tighter and tighter! OK, let go! Relax your hand and arm. Relax and let the tension drain away. Let yourself experience fully how relaxed and good your hand and arm now feels.

   This time tighten the muscles in your right foot and leg. Squeeze and contract them as hard as you can. When they are very tight let them go and relax. Concentrate on the good feelings of release in your foot and leg.

   Now tighten the muscles in your left foot and leg. Make them as tight as you possibly can, so tight that you can actually feel the entire lower left side of your body tensing up, then relax, let go, and feel that tension draining away.

   Shift your attention to your shoulders and neck muscles. Slowly tense them up. Now shrug your shoulders, tighten them up, and clench both fists and tighten both of your arms and your entire torso. Feel how tight it is becoming, tighter and tighter! OK, let go and relax! First your neck, then your shoulders, your arms, your hands, your entire torso. Concentrate on how good it feels to drain off all of that tension as you relax and let go.

   Now get a picture of yourself in your mind as you begin to tighten your entire body. Yes, your entire body is beginning to get tense. First your feet and legs–make them tense and rigid as before. Now clench both fists and tighten your arms. Now tighten your neck and shoulders, and now bend over a bit and begin to make your entire body into one tight and tense ball, tighter, tighter!

continued

Now relax, relax and let go all over. Think of the tension draining off from your feet and legs, from your hands and arms, from your neck and shoulders, tension draining from your entire body. As it drains and as you relax your muscles even more, you feel so good–much better in fact than you have for some time. You feel good and deeply relaxed and your entire body feels refreshed.

2. **Body Awareness.** As you continue to relax yourself, place your hands in your lap with your right hand resting lightly on your left hand. Now concentrate your attention on your hands. Do not move them but become aware of the texture of the skin beneath your fingers. Feel the warmth of your skin. Think of the pressure of your fingers on your hand, the pressure of your hands on your lap.

You can now become aware of the texture of your clothes under your hand. Feel the clothes pressing against your body. Concentrate on the pressure of your feet and your shoes against the floor.

Now shift your attention to your skin. You are actually becoming aware of the skin on parts of your body. You feel very good and very relaxed as you become increasingly aware of your body and the life energy within you. Now you can feel that energy moving through your entire body, circulating and nourishing your body and entire self. As you relax and concentrate you can become aware of your pulse beat. Faintly in your awareness you can feel it beat stronger as you concentrate on it. As you relax and concentrate you can feel your heart pumping your blood and refreshing your body and mind.

Now as you begin to concentrate on your heart beat you relax yourself even more. Let yourself become even more deeply relaxed. You are now aware of your entire body relaxing and working in beautiful harmony. You can feel yourself and your body energy moving harmoniously to an even deeper stage of relaxation and you feel good all over.

3. **Breathing.** Just continue to sit quietly and enjoy your sense of deep relaxation. Let your mind and body be quiet and relaxed. As you let yourself become more relaxed you will begin to breathe more deeply. Gradually, you will begin to take deeper and deeper breaths. That's it! Deeper and slower, deeper and slower–even more relaxed.

As you become increasingly aware of your deep breathing you will feel even better throughout your entire body. Now just concentrate on your breathing. Slowly you inhale, then even more slowly and deeply exhale. As you exhale you feel your chest and your stomach becoming more relaxed. As the rhythm of your deep breathing becomes steady you can feel your hands slowly rising and falling on your lap or abdomen.

You feel good, very good! Let yourself concentrate even more fully on your deep rhythmic breathing. Now begin to slowly count each exhalation of breath and as you do so, relax yourself even more deeply. Good! Just count and let yourself relax more deeply.

continued

Fine! You are deeply relaxed but you are not sleepy and you are acutely aware of yourself and the good feeling of your deep breathing. Attend carefully to the feeling of air expanding in your lungs as you inhale. It is truly the breath of universal life that is entering and energizing your entire mind and body. Now concentrate on your exhalations and as you count them again let yourself continue to become deeply and soundly relaxed. That's the way! Count the exhalations and relax. Deeper and deeper. How good you feel as you let yourself go and become deeply in touch with your self.

4. **Focusing Self-Energy.** Now you will stop counting your exhalations of breath and just relax quietly. As you do so be sure that the palms and fingers of your hands are resting lightly against your abdomen. And as you continue to breathe deeply, again focus your attention on the slow rise and fall of your abdomen. You are aware of the rhythmic rise and fall of your abdomen through your hands and fingers and other parts of your body as well. It is a very deeply relaxing sensation.

As you focus your attention on your abdomen you will gradually become aware of the great energy that lies within you and is coursing through and nourishing your body. This energy has been activated through your deeply relaxed breathing and the harmonious workings of your body and mind.

Your self-energy is now concentrated in your abdomen. Relax and let yourself feel it. It is centered just below your navel and as you continue your deep rhythmic breathing, focus all of your attention on this part of your body. As you do so you will experience a pleasant warmth emanating from the center of your abdomen.

It begins to feel as though your abdomen has been warmed by the rays of the sun or by a heating pad. Let yourself experience this pleasant warmth. Deep within you, your body energy is centering in this part of your self. It feels very good and relaxing and is energizing and restoring your entire system.

Now as you continue to focus your attention on this center of emanating warmth and energy, it slowly, so very, very slowly, begins to move up through your torso. As it moves, continue to breathe deeply and experience the warmth and great feeling of rejuvenation that is spreading through your entire body.

You now feel very good and your center of energy is moving on up through your chest and the pleasant warmth makes your breathing even more easy and relaxed. The center of energy is now in the middle of your chest right between your breasts. Focus on it and feel the rays of energy slowly spread out from it.

continued

Remain quiet and continue to focus on the center of your chest and visualize the glowing warmth and let yourself experience the emanating energy that is spreading throughout your chest, down your arms, upward to your head, and is now beginning to cover your entire body.

Relax, center yourself and enjoy this good feeling of nourishment and energy. Listen to your own breathing as you visualize this center of energy in your chest that is continuing to warm and relax you. Let yourself feel the rays of energy as they move out to parts of your body and as you visualize them in your mind. Identify yourself with this center of energy and give yourself to it for a moment as you continue to relax.

5. **Visualization.** You now feel very good indeed as you continue to relax yourself and focus on your center of energy and being. This center is beginning to shift again. Slowly it moves up through the back of your chest, to your neck. As it does so, your back and neck become pleasantly warm and relaxed. Now it continues to move up through your neck and across the back of your head and it feels very good. Slowly now, your center of self-energy moves down from the crown of your head to your forehead and then comes to rest at the center point between your eyes.

Let yourself remain very relaxed and focus your attention on the point between your eyes. In your mind you can see and feel the pleasant glow and warmth from this centering of your energy. This centering point will now begin to change itself into a mental picture of a brightly glowing full moon. As you relax you can begin to picture this round, full moon very clearly.

Picture yourself sitting comfortably by a quiet and soothing lake bathed in the moonlight. The waters beneath the moon ripple gently and with a mild breeze stirring you feel very tranquil and at peace with yourself. Feel the breeze and enjoy the beautiful shimmering of the light reflected in the water.

As you focus on this pleasant scene you begin to merge yourself with it. You gradually become one with the moon, and the mild breeze, and the peaceful water. You feel relaxed, whole and one with nature and yourself. Now you relax and enjoy the feeling of wholeness, of unity, of oneness and you feel good all over.

Slowly now the scene changes again. The moon begins to fade away into the dawn of a new day. The rays of the sun are apparent on the horizon and you can feel the joy and anticipation of the new day about to be born. As the sun rises, you can feel your energy stirring within you and your body is warm and comfortable and vigorously alive. Now the sun is up and a few white and beautiful clouds are forming, and slowly they begin to move across the sky. A slight breeze comes up and stirs and refreshes you as it moves over your body. You feel so refreshed and renewed and you too begin to eagerly anticipate meeting the new day before you.

continued

In a moment now the scene will begin to fade away and your eyes will slowly open but you will continue to feel relaxed and refreshed. Now it is time; the scene is fading and now it is gone, but you can still feel the freshness of the breeze and the warmth within you. Open your eyes and look about you and remain aware of how good you feel. Stretch out your arms and hands and prepare to encounter the day. Now stand and stretch and hug yourself with vigor and enthusiasm. This day is yours and will be what you make it. Go now and live it with contentment and a sense of well-being until you wish to return again to this time of self-relaxation, centering, and self-renewal.

Evaluation: Check ability to relax and follow each exercise.

Exercise	Poor	Fair	Good
1. Tensing			
2. Body awareness			
3. Breathing			
4. Focusing self-energy			
5. Visualization			

Variations: Use a tape recorder to tape students' own voices giving themselves these exercises. Try other kinds of relaxation exercises such as yoga positions.

MOTIVATION AND REINFORCEMENT

If anxiety levels and stress reactions to reading are reduced, the dyslexic child will be more capable of focusing and maintaining his or her attention. However, some learning tasks and reading programs are much more interesting and rewarding to children than others. To be effective, reading tasks must be both intrinsically and extrinsically rewarding. That is, the child must have personal involvement and interest in (intrinsic) and derive satisfaction from (extrinsic) the "instructional encounter" with the teacher.

For example, developmental or remedial programs that require creative imagination and actively involve the student are usually much more successful than nonimaginative ones. Colin Wilson (1972) concludes that the greatest of all aids to concentration is imagnation. Personal growth is enhanced by an active creative imagination that aspires to a more positive self-image and accomplishment. Much of the pioneer work of David McClelland (1953) and his associates on the development of achievement motivation involves the creative use of materials, toys, and games to spark the interest of students. Intrinsic motivation is essentially self-motivation that grows out of successfully accomplishing interesting and meaningful tasks. Intrinsic motivation is germinated by appropriate reading tasks and assignments that are also novel, challenging, and relevant to the child's developmental stage. When playfulness, humor, creative imagination, and increasing self-direction are provided in the instructional program, motivation and achievement are furthered.

Much has been written on the use of behavior modification techniques to provide extrinsic motivation in the classroom. Rewards, such as praise, social privileges, and tokens to be exchanged for desired goods or activities, encourage the dyslexic child to attend to and accomplish his or her prescriptive reading task. Many positive reinforcement systems and methods for use by both teachers and parents are presented by Valett (1969, 1970, 1977) and others. Schaefer (1977) gives a recent summary of research on methods for improving intrinsic and extrinsic motivation in underachieving children.

As an example of an imaginative and highly motivating approach to reading let us consider the use of fairy tales. Bettelheim (1975) believes that fairy tales stimulate a child's imagination, help to develop intellect, and clarify emotions. Fairy tales hold the child's attention and arouse curiosity if they are carefully selected and attuned to both the child's anxieties and aspirations. A good fairy tale will also suggest some possible solutions to the problems confronting the child.

Bettelheim explains how the fairy tale is the primer from which the child can learn to read his or her own mind in the language of visual and verbal images. In this way, the fantasy life of the child can be encountered in reality and the intrinsic motivating powers of his or her imagination can be put to work to further development. It is preferable to tell (or retell) fairy tales at first rather than to read them, because this allows greater flexibility. Fairy tales can then be read, reread, acted out, and supplemented in many different ways to increase motivation and involvement. Some of the most useful fairy tales are listed here:

- Cinderella
- The Emperor's New Clothes
- Jack and the Bean Stalk
- Three Little Pigs
- The Ugly Duckling
- The Frog Prince
- Hansel and Gretel
- Beauty and the Beast

It takes a skilled and mature teacher to be able to use dreams or fairy tales constructively. However, through the means of dramatics, puppets, dreams, and creative writing, children can be motivated to take part in the story-making and reading processes.

Such participation can improve students' self-esteem. Pine (1977) compared six traditional first-grade classrooms to six activity-centered classrooms (some 257 children). No significant differences in reading achievement scores were found, but self-concepts and motivation in the activity-centered classes were significantly higher. Several years ago Parker (1957) demonstrated positive changes in the self-esteem and motivation of college students brought about by the use of creative imagination and positive visualization activities. A recent report on the place of the arts in education cites programs that integrated creative art activities with basic instruction and improved reading performance at twice the normal rate (Sanders 1977).

In a collection of readings on the nature of human consciousness, Ornstein (1973) discusses several possibilities for increasing motivation and learning. Ornstein describes how the unique functions of the right and left hemispheres of the human brain should be tapped and integrated through the use of creative and imaginative educational programs. This education of the intuitive-imaginative-creative mode should involve psychological self-mastery, body energies, death confrontation, dream experiences, and other expressive forms. It has also been proposed that report cards in the future be modified to include grades for such right-brain functions as spatial relationships, insight, intuition, imagination, fantasy, empathy, transcendence, and self-evaluation (Brain/Mind Bulletin 1975).

Schools that have developmental programs tend to use report cards that stress continuous individual growth in many different important areas of human development. One example is the Human Development Report Card shown on page 200. For dyslexic children, it is especially important that the skills beyond the first group shown on the card be recognized and rewarded.

An exercise in motivation and reinforcement follows on page 201.

BEHAVIORAL PROGRAMMING

Luria (1973) explains how arousal and attention are part of the regulatory brain unit. When a person has focused his or her attention on a learning task, there are distinctive physiological correlates. The first stage of coming to attention is largely an orienting reaction to directive stimuli, such as a teacher's instruction. Then the person begins to focus on selected stimuli relevant to the immediate situation (such as a dyslexic child beginning to focus on specific medial consonant sounds or blends in words). Finally, the problem is one of maintaining or continuing the focus over a period of time. This focusing requires screening out irrelevant noise or other distracting stimuli. This process of directivity, selectivity, and organization of mental processing abilities is "attention."

Luria's work also shows how the frontal lobes play an important role in raising the level of vigilance and thus participate in higher forms of attention. In the beginning, attention to task may result from socially focused, organized directions from a child's parent or teacher. Eventually, though, voluntary self-regulated attention should begin to develop. For the person with basic neuropsychological disturbances, the initial orientation reaction to stimuli can be made easier and focused attention can be improved through the use of self-verbalization

HUMAN DEVELOPMENT REPORT CARD

Name   Age   School

	Superior Development A	Well-Developed B	Being Developed C	Under-Developed D	Un-Developed F
Thinking Skills					
Reading					
Writing					
Arithmetic					
Spelling					
Speaking					
Other:					
Sensing Skills					
Attention and concentration					
Listening and following directions					
Spatial organization					
Art and drawing					
Rhythm/dancing					
Music					
Body skills/sports/games					
Feeling Skills					
Emotional expression					
Cooperation					
Empathy					
Value orientation/ethics					
Self-control					
Social responsibility					
Intuiting Skills					
Imagination					
Creativity					
Inventiveness					
Foresight					
Insight					
Transcendence					
Self-actualization					

Objective: to use and channel fantasy and imagination

Materials: tape recorder, paper, crayons

Directions: Put your head in your arms on your desk and relax. I want you to imagine that you are a little bear. Close your eyes and picture how you would look, how you walk, and how you feel:

1. Imagine what it is like to be a little bear. Picture where you have been, what has happened to you, and where you are going.

2. Now winter is coming. You are going into a special place to hibernate and sleep until spring.

3. Imagine that the snow is melting. Spring has finally arrived and you are waking up and leaving your cave. How do you feel and act? Imagine and make up a story in your mind about where you will go and what will happen to you.

4. Now sit up, open your eyes, and tell me all that you imagined while you were a bear. We will tape-record your story.

5. Make a colored picture of your bear story.

6. Listen to your recorded story. As you listen to the story try to feel and act like a bear again. Move about the room and show me what you would be doing.

7. On the bottom of your picture write a sentence or very short story about your bear. If you need help with spelling let me know and I will help you.

Evaluation:

	+	+ /-	-	Comments
Verbalization				
Enactment				
Drawing				
Writing				

Variations: Have the child tell the story to another student. Use fairy tales and dreams, asking the children to tell them, enact them, and finally write out part of his or her fantasy.

procedures, such as thinking aloud or talking to oneself. This form of self-instruction appears to initiate frontal-lobe involvement that triggers other neurophysiological mechanisms needed to attend and concentrate.

An early study by Walters and Doan (1962) on the perceptual and cognitive functioning deficiencies of retarded readers shows that these children have significant difficulty in focusing on and attending to verbal symbols. However, reinforcement and contingency management programs proved to be highly effective in remediating these problems. Since then many studies have shown the superiority of behavioral programming and reinforcement methods with dyslexic children.

The effect of differential reinforcement schedules on inattentive hyperactive learning-disabled children has been researched in detail. Meichenbaum (1976) argues for a psychoeducational analysis of the cognitive requirements in reading tasks. Such requirements can then be behaviorally programmed. For example, attention to highly specific sounds could be structured and shaped through appropriate reinforcement techniques. Tarver (1976) and his colleagues conducted a study of selective attention in learning-disabled children and found their major deficiencies to be in strategies for repetition, rehearsal, guided practice, and self-reinforcement. They also found that verbal rehearsal and reinforcement programs facilitate the development of these critical strategies. A study by Parry (1973) suggests that immediate praise is the most effective reinforcement for improving attention in hyperactive learning-disabled children and that the use of random reinforcement actually weakens inhibitory control and distracts students. Several applied research studies combine some of these techniques into programs for reading-disabled children.

Staats and Butterfield (1965) used a behavioral reinforcement program with a fourteen-year-old nonreading juvenile delinquent. The boy had a poor attention span, showed poorly integrated thought processes, was performing on the second-grade level, and was failing in school. However, he was found to be of normal intelligence with good conventional judgment. A token economy was devised whereby the tokens could be exchanged for such things as phonograph records, ice cream, and tickets to special events. The remedial reading program emphasized sight word vocabulary, oral paragraph and short story reading, and the incidental sounding out of words. With systematic reinforcement, the child improved his reading performance to the high third-grade level in only forty hours of instruction.

McCormick and Poetker (1968) were among the first to

demonstrate that Luria's attention training procedures improved reading. Moyer and Newcomer (1977) review extensive research showing how specific behavioral instruction and discrimination training can be used to eliminate reversals of letters and words in young children. Friedman, Guyer-Christie, and Tymchuk (1976) say verbal and attentional skills are both left-hemispheric functions that are enhanced through imagery training and self-verbalization strategies. Billingsley (1977) shows that reading improves when children are allowed to choose the number of words to be read aloud. Similarly, Bender (1976) reports studies on the use of self-verbalization as against tutor verbalization in modifying impulsivity of children in classroom settings. Students taught verbal self-instruction techniques proved superior to control groups on criterion tests.

There are several behavioral programs for improving attention in learning-disabled children that can be adapted for classroom use. Connor (1974) published a booklet of individual and group classroom activities useful in reducing hyperactivity and increasing attention. Valett (1974) wrote a prescriptive psychoeducational treatment program manual for use with hyperactive and inattentive learning-disabled children that includes material for self-evaluation and parent involvement. A copy of the Parent and Teacher Rating Scale for Hyperactive Behavior from Valett's manual is reproduced on the next two pages.

Fagen, Nicholas, and Stevens (1975) have designed educational strategies and school programs for teaching self-control skills as part of the elementary school curriculum. The essence of most good behavioral program strategies for use with dyslexic and learning-disabled children can be summarized as follows:

1. Analyze deficiencies in the child's ability to pay attention and process symbolic information.

2. Select appropriate learning tasks and highly motivating reinforcers.

3. Have the child demonstrate understanding of task instructions through self-verbalization before, during, and after the task.

4. Require students to record their progress and evaluate their work.

5. Follow up on the retention of information or skills. Use further rehearsal and self-directive practice lessons with continued reinforcement.

An exercise in behavioral programming follows.

PARENT AND TEACHER RATING SCALE FOR HYPERACTIVE BEHAVIOR

Child's Name _____ Rater's Name _____

Dates of Rating: Parent (Black X) _____ Teacher (Red X) _____

Directions: Please rate this child on each of the behaviors described below. Place an X mark in the box on the scale that indicates your estimate of the child's behavior compared to other "normal" children of the same age and sex. Then write in an example of the behavior you have observed.

Behavior to Be Rated	Less Than Most Children	Just Like Most Others	Slightly More Than Most	More Than Most	Much More Than Most	Very Much More Than Most
	0	1	2	3	4	5

1. **Excessive Body Movement** constant over-activity: squirming, moving, walking, throwing, and so forth

   Example:

2. **Impulsiveness** frequently acts and moves on spur of the moment without thinking of results

   Example:

3. **Poor Attention Span** does not pay attention to, concentrate on, or complete assignments or projects

   Example:

4. **Inconsistency** wide unpredictable variations in behavior and performance

   Example:

5. **Emotionality** has explosive temper tantrums and other emotional outbreaks

   Example:

continued

6. **Poor Visual-Motor Coordination**   difficulty in writing, drawing, tracing, cutting, and so forth

   Example:

7. **Arithmetic Difficulties**   problems in accuracy and in doing addition, subtraction, multiplication, division, and so forth

   Example:

8. **Poor Reading**   problems in associating alphabet sounds and letters, phonics, comprehension, and so forth

   Example:

9. **Poor Memory**   easily forgets instructions, directions, lessons, assignments, and so forth

   Example:

10. **Failure Prone**   tends to give up quickly; reluctant to attempt new tasks

    Example:

Comments:

Parent's Rating Total: _____

Teacher's Rating Total: _____

Combined Total: _____

Objective: to concentrate on and follow sequential symbolic information

Materials: worksheet

Directions: Look carefully at the worksheet that I will give you. Begin on line number 1 and put your pencil on each symbol as I name them in order. When I say a symbol that is **not** the one you see, draw a circle around yours with your pencil. Each line has one incorrect symbol. (The teacher should substitute another symbol for those in parenthesis on the sample worksheet below.)

1.	a	9	7	in	(O)	2	boy	10	t	5
2.	t	c	(1)	m	girl	v	8	L	b	3
3.	m	g	man	c	(6)	q	r	4	b	8
4.	w	1	3	g	u	(up)	7	b	e	x
5.	x	–	(e)	4	f	v	cat	10	O	c
6.	d	c	s	n	2	5	p	(8)	out	r
7.	i	4	p	t	y	7	n	a	2	(ball)
8.	b	(1)	horse	h	+	u	j	5	k	9
9.	run	k	h	(2)	m	10	3	X	2	7
10.	k	eat	y	s	a	7	+	c	(f)	5

Evaluation: Number of errors _____

Time _____

Variations: Repeat lessons with teacher reading symbols faster. Have student maintain a record of several trials. Have students write or design their own worksheets.

NUTRITION AND DRUG MANAGEMENT

Another way to increase attention and concentration in dyslexic children is through drug and nutrition programs. Stimulant medications such as dextroamphetamine and methylphenidate have long been administered to hyperactive and learning-disabled children. (The reader may be interested in these special reports: a special issue of the *Journal of Learning Disabilities,* Volume 4, Number 9, 1971, entitled "The Role of Medication in the Treatment of Learning Disabilities and Related Behavior Disorders"; and *The School Psychology Digest,* Volume 5, Number 4, 1976.)

It is extremely important for special educators to understand the rationale underlying drug management and how such treatment may affect reading performance. Most dyslexic children suffer from biochemical and metabolic dysfunctions that interfere with focused attention and the normal processing and integration of neural impulses. Medication (in the proper dosage) may be needed to restore biochemical balance. Pribam and McGuiness (1975) describe how serotonergic compounds (such as epinephrine and L-dopa) activate the inhibitory mechanisms in the medial hypothalamic areas and help to screen extraneous noise and focus attention. Wender (1976) explains how genetic dysfunction can interfere with the production of neurotransmitters, such as serotonin, and how stimulant drugs cause cells to release the biochemicals required in attention processes. As an example, amphetamine may help focus arousal and enable the child to fix and maintain attention.

Dr. Lendon Smith has written a book for parents explaining how they may improve their children's behavior through proper diet and medical care. Smith states that the lack of the stimulant norepinephrine in the limbic or reticular activating system is as critical for a learning-disabled child as the lack of insulin is for a diabetic. He further states that the cortex must be "made alert and receptive by diet, vitamins, medicine, alpha awareness, motivation, and/or love" (Smith 1976, p. 156).

Other researchers, such as Cott (1972) and Rimland (1973), report that high dosages of vitamins (B, C, B_6, niacinamide) increase alertness and social awareness in handicapped children. Feingold (1975) presents controversial research advocating a salicylate-free diet to reduce allergic predispositions and reactions in distractible and impulsive children. Other kinds of biochemical dysfunctions, such as thyroid disorders and their effect on dyslexic children, are considered by Park and Schneider (1975) and others.

The study by Conners, Rothschild, Eisenberg, Schwartz, and Robinson (1969) on the effect of dextroamphetamine sulfate on the perception, learning, and achievement of learning-disabled children has become a classic reference. Forty-five learning-disabled elementary-school children were given an average of 25 milligrams of dextroamphetamine sulfate daily for four weeks. They improved in arithmetic achievement tests, rote learning, auditory synthesis tasks, and visual perception tests. Some improvement ($p < .10$ level) was obtained on the Wide Range Reading test. The only adverse side effects were loss of appetite or sleep in some children, which called for a decrease in dosage. Similar studies have been done by Gittelman-Klein (1975) and by Lerer and Lerer (1977) using methylphenidate (Ritalin). They report improvement in visual-motor functions, concentration and attention, school grades, and achievement test scores.

Some research has been conducted on the effects of motion sickness medication on dyslexic children. Frank and Levinson (1975–76) define dyslexia as a cerebellar-vestibular dysfunction resulting in subclinical nystagmus and problems in ocular fixation. They recommend motion sickness medication be used along with drugs such as Ritalin, cerebellar-vestibular exercises (Ayres 1972), and controlled phrase reading. Later these same investigators studied 280 dysmetric-dyslexic cases (Frank and Levinson 1977) who were treated with motion sickness medication (Marezine, Antivert, Dramamine) over a three-month period. A third of this group reportedly showed "dramatic improvement" in spatial orientation, attention, reversals, writing, balance, and coordination. The improvement was attributed to the medication serving as "cerebellar-vestibular harmonizing agents." It must be stated that the Frank and Levinson studies were poorly designed and have not been validated. Clinical evidence still suggests that medication may affect the vestibular system and improve focused awareness and attention in dyslexic children.

Considered as a whole, the evidence is overwhelming that many inattentive, distractible dyslexic children could profit from appropriate medication and improved diet. Oettinger (1978) says that about 75 percent of learning-disabled children profiting from medication may have to remain on it throughout most of their lives. However, medication does not take the place of prescriptive teaching and other forms of educational treatment. These must come first. With dyslexic and highly inattentive children, it is essential that the special educator work closely with the child's physician, parents, and other psychoeducational specialists.

PARENT SUPPORT

Parents can do much to reduce children's anxieties, improve their attention spans, increase their motivation for reading, and support them in the continued development of good reading skills. Bronfenbrenner (1974) reviews the effect of a child's family on his or her achievement in later life and cites the earlier findings of James Coleman, who studied six hundred thousand children in all grades. Home background is the most important element in determining how well a child will do in school. Especially important is the parent's positive attitude toward learning, and the presence and use of books and other reading materials in the home.

Many educational institutions and publishing firms have promoted reading in the home and have provided parents with instructional guides and materials (Scholastic Magazine, undated). Some of these special programs for parents have been very systematically organized. Radin (1969) organized a home training program for parents of preschool children. In one year children of these parents made twice the gain of control children on the reading readiness subtest of the Metropolitan Achievement Test. Early parent involvement in verbalization and cognitive development tasks produced the largest gains. Another similar study by Smith (1968) involved one thousand black low-income families in a home-school program in which parents read aloud to children, listened to children read, read quietly in the presence of their children, and gave encouragement and praise for reading. Second and fifth-grade students made significant gains in reading achievement in this program, and it was found that *supportive* parent help (not directive teaching) produced the most significant results.

Several popular books have been written by parents of learning-handicapped children to explain how other parents may be helpful and supportive. Especially recommended is *Can't Read, Can't Write, Can't Talk Too Good Either* by Louise Clarke, the mother of a dyslexic boy. Books of this sort can be used by professionals as examples for parents and classroom teachers.

Special educators should provide parent education and counseling

1. Take the time to listen to your children as much as you can (really try to get their "message").

2. Love them by touching them, hugging them, tickling them, wrestling with them (they need lots of physical contact).

3. Look for and encourage their strengths, interests, and abilities. Help them to use these as compensations for any limitations or disabilities.

4. Reward them with praise, good words, smiles, and a pat on the back as often as you can.

5. Accept them for what they are and for their human potential for growth and development. Be realistic in your expectations and demands.

6. Involve them in establishing rules and regulations, schedules, and family activities.

7. Tell them when they misbehave and explain how you feel about their behavior; then have them propose other, more acceptable ways of behaving.

8. Help them to correct their errors and mistakes by showing or demonstrating what they should do. Don't nag!

9. Use force and spanking only when absolutely necessary and then be sure to follow it immediately with corrective guidance.

10. Give them reasonable chores and a regular family work responsibility whenever possible.

11. Give them an allowance as early as possible and then help them plan to spend within it.

12. Provide toys, games, motor activities, and opportunities that will stimulate them in their development.

13. Read enjoyable stories to them and with them. Encourage them to ask questions, discuss stories, tell the story, and to reread stories.

14. Further their ability to concentrate by reducing distracting aspects of their environment as much as possible (provide them with a place to work, study, and play).

15. Don't get hung up on traditional school grades! It is important that they progress at their own rates and be rewarded for doing so.

16. Take them to libraries and encourage them to select and check out books of interest. Have them share their books with you. Provide stimulating books and reading material around the house.

17. Help them to develop self-esteem and to compete with self rather than with others.

18. Insist that they cooperate socially by playing, helping, and serving others in the family and the community.

19. Serve as a model to them by reading and discussing material of personal interest. Share with them some of the things you are reading and doing.

20. Don't hesitate to consult with teachers or other specialists whenever you feel it to be necessary in order to better understand what might be done to help your child learn.

programs to enable the parents of dyslexic children to help their children more effectively. The preceding list of twenty suggestions has been found useful by special educators when conferring with and counseling parents or in parent education programs. It is most helpful when used with a cooperative home and school diagnostic-prescriptive education program.

SUMMARY
There are several ways to help dyslexic children improve their attention and motivation for learning. The first of these is to understand the dynamics of attention and its neuropsychological basis. Relaxation, meditation, and self-suggestion can be taught and may reduce anxiety levels in dyslexics. Highly motivating lessons and programs using the child's imagination, interesting stories, and movement activities also help to increase attention and learning. Behavioral programming and positive reinforcement should be used with dyslexic children. Also, proper medication may result in sustained attention and make the child more amenable to remedial or developmental instruction.

Parents are the cornerstone of any special education program for dyslexic children. With their involvement and support in modeling attentive behavior and through the use of home training programs, the dyslexic child can continue to make significant progress in learning to read.

DISCUSSION QUESTIONS AND ACTIVITIES

1. Discuss how anxiety interferes with reading performance.
2. What study shows that meditation can improve auditory-perceptual discrimination and memory?
3. Use relaxation and suggestion exercises with a dyslexic child and report your results.
4. What is unique about Jampolsky's training program?
5. Demonstrate the use of selected yoga techniques to improve attention in children.
6. Discuss how intrinsic motivation may be acquired.
7. Use a fairy tale or dream lesson with a reading-disabled child and evaluate your results.

8. Devise a report card for marking progress in the development of total brain functions (both hemispheres).

9. What is the Vygotsky-Luria approach to the remediation of attention deficiencies?

10. Create a self-evaluation or self-regulatory reading lesson for a dyslexic child.

11. When should medication be used with dyslexic children? Why?

12. Discuss the Frank and Levinson studies.

13. What is the most significant factor in determining how well a child will achieve in school?

Whatever you cannot understand,
you cannot possess.

Goethe

CHAPTER ELEVEN

Developing Reading Comprehension

Reading comprehension involves much more than the acquisition of such fundamental skills as phonetics and the mechanics of language. True comprehension is also dependent upon the development of cognitive structures and operations that emerge from the interaction of maturation and appropriate education. In this chapter we will consider some of these factors and their importance in educating dyslexic children.

SET AND EXPECTATION

If we want dyslexic children to improve in comprehension of what they read, we need to begin with an evaluation of their current reading performance. Can the child read sentences and story paragraphs (both silently and aloud) and interpret them accurately as evidenced by his or her answers to content questions? Can the child follow story directions or paraphrase the theme or plot?

In order to accomplish such tasks, the child must have acquired certain listening and thinking skills. A teacher must take into account the child's developmental stage and assign reading tasks that are neither too easy nor too difficult and that stimulate the student. This is especially important for dyslexic children.

One approach to the evaluation of cognitive skills required in reading comprehension is through the use of tests such as the verbal opposites section of the Detroit Test of Learning Aptitude. The verbal opposites test is very useful in determining a child's reading comprehension and potential. This test can be used separately or as part of the broader diagnostic battery described in Chapter 5. First, the teacher tells the child a word (boy, up, off, strong) from the verbal opposites word list and asks for the opposite (for example, boy: girl; up: down). Mental age scores (which are really *word comprehension age* scores) are then derived from the oral responses. Next, the child is asked to read each word from the list aloud, give its opposite, and use it in a sentence. The word comprehension age score is then noted and contrasted with the first score to determine discrepancy and reading potential. As a check on dysgraphic tendencies and spelling and auditory decoding difficulties, it is usually helpful to have dyslexic persons take the test yet a third time, this time reading the word and writing its opposite. Scores from functional reading comprehension tests help place the child at an appropriate developmental reading level. Responses to such tests can also be used directly in prescriptive programming.

Good prescriptive programming begins with a consideration of motivation. Skinner (1965) believes that good teachers arrange contingencies to reinforce learning in students. He reminds us that "good books" are those that stimulate the reader by giving pleasure. Reading should be reinforced by choosing material in which the child displays interest, for only then will the reward of reading—understanding—bring pleasure.

A review of recent studies by Algozzine and Sutherland (1977) concludes that most learning-disabled children are not actually disabled but disinterested. These researchers argue that the structure of the learning environment in most schools produces disinterest and apathy. Dyslexic children must have a well-designed and organized individual instructional program (an Individual Educational Plan—IEP) that includes highly motivating and appropriate material if reading comprehension is to be successfully developed.

Spector (1978) describes a neuropsychological test approach—based on the Halstead-Reitan test battery—to the diagnosis and remediation of specific cognitive deficiencies in dyslexic children. Several years ago Reitan (1955) found that left-hemispheric lesions are associated with lower verbal scores than performance scores on the Wechsler tests, while right-hemispheric or diffused damage resulted in lower performance scores. Spector uses prescriptive tasks with dyslexic children to develop cognitive operations and hemispheric integration, thus contributing to the improvement of general comprehension and reading performance.

Ashton-Warner (1963) observes that children improve their comprehension when reading material uses culturally relevant words that express their own concerns and feelings. For example, *ghost* is a highly motivating word with particular relevance for certain cultural groups. The use of that word stimulates feelings, involvement, and comprehension. We have discussed how emotional expression through fairy tale and dream enactment can be helpful. Educational television programs, such as "Sesame Street," "The Electric Company," and "Mr. Rogers's Neighborhood," use fantasy well. For instance, the strategy of "The Electric Company" is to stimulate reading through the use of fantasy characters named "Easy Reader" and "Fargo North, Decoder." These shows have proved highly successful in reaching nonreading children and involving them in a reading process that is meaningful and comprehensible.

Linguistic approaches are also used with disabled readers. Structural linguistic materials first help the child to break the code by using in printed form the words and sentences he or she already uses and understands in daily speech. They systematically help the child to identify the distinctive features of spoken and written language through a single method of word attack and controlled vocabulary. Some studies show that children can learn to read and understand five thousand different words in eighteen months and are then able to engage in more critical and thoughtful reading (Fishbein 1967). One example of this kind of pragmatic material is the Sullivan Programmed Reading series of twenty-one sequential workbooks that have long been used with reading-handicapped children. Structural linguistic material by itself, though, is insufficient to develop reading comprehension.

Most developmental-remedial reading programs use varied materials and techniques to improve reading comprehension. One frequently used technique is having the child dictate short paragraphs and stories using a tape recorder. These stories are then typed by the teacher, parent, or aides, and the vocabulary is taught within the context of the child's syntax and functional comprehension. One such study by Smith, Adams, Schomer, and Willardson (1971) shows that an experimental group of second-grade children, as compared to controls, made significant gains in paragraph meaning subtest scores on the reading achievement section of the Stanford Diagnostic Reading Test. Many of these techniques have been systematically developed and produced commercially, for example the Leir Language Experience in Reading Program by Van Allen and Venezky.

Other more traditional approaches are summarized by Roswell and Natchez (1977). These include developing reading comprehension by teaching children such skills as skimming a story or book, underlining, reviewing, questioning, understanding sentence context and semantic analysis, and carefully studying vocabulary meanings reflected in prefixes, suffixes, and root words.

At the end of this chapter there are several exercises covering differing aspects of reading comprehension.

A COGNITIVE TAXONOMY

Reading comprehension depends on the development of general intelligence and such basic mental abilities as serial thinking, classification, and analogous thought. The retarded child obviously has much more difficulty understanding abstract words and relationships than a child of average or superior general learning ability. Early studies by Coleman (1953) and by Walters and Doan (1962) show that retarded readers have great difficulty in making perceptual discriminations of symbolic material (especially verbal symbols) because of higher-order cognitive dysfunction. However, we now know that specific symbolic learning tasks (such as "seeing" relationships in figures, understanding similarities, and so forth) can also be systematically developed through proper prescriptive education and reinforcement.

For dyslexic children with neuropsychological dysfunctions in the programming brain unit, "short circuiting" in the frontal lobes will interfere with conscious thinking, feedback, and symbolic learning. Since the programming brain unit is also concerned with planning and synthesis of information, developmental-remedial lessons may be necessary in specific cognitive operations.

Considerable work has been done on the prescriptive development of cognitive abilities. Most special educators are aware of the contributions of Inhelder and Piaget (1958), Guilford (1967), and others who have presented models of intellectual abilities and operations that can be influenced by education. Bloom (1956) and his colleagues developed a classification of cognitive objectives that has long been used by teachers of all kinds. Recently, Valett compiled a review of research and methodologies that deal with the development of cognitive abilities in young children with learning problems. Table 6, attempts a synthesis of available models that are currently used in special education.

TABLE 6. Cognitive Skills Instructional Taxonomy*

Cognitive objectives	Sensory-motor adaptations (birth to 2 years)	Preoperational intuitions (2 to 7 years)	Concrete manipulations (7 to 11 years)	Formal reversible operations (11 years and older)
Knowledge: conditioned responses, terms, facts, conventions, methods, classes, and relations	Reflexive assimilations, visual-motor accommodations, schematic organizations and coordination	Perceptual-representative judgment, irreversibility, intuitional abstractions	Receptive vocabulary, general information, number concepts	
Comprehension: elements, rules, translation, interpretation, extrapolation	Experimental discovery	Single property classification, correspondence of sets, visual generalizations, simple seriation	Seriation of pictures and patterns, quantitative seriation, conservation of quantity and space, arithmetic computation, multiple classification, reading vocabulary, general comprehension	Time, reversibility
Application: Semantic, figural, symbolic, behavioral	Invention	Manual expression, perceptual-motor coordination, visual-motor memory	Mathematical reasoning, language mechanics, expressive vocabulary	Reality problem solving, creative divergency, social competency
Analysis: Units, relationships, organizational principles	Listening and attending, visual organization and closure		Auditory-vocal sequential memory, word-attack skills, spelling, reference skills	Propositional thinking
Synthesis: Integration, planning, originality, theorizing	Motor planning, visual-motor patterns, visual-motor integration		Sensory integration, auditory vocal closure, reading comprehension, similarities	Figural-symbolic abstractions and relationships
Evaluation: self-criticism, external validation, implications	Self-awareness		Analogies, social interpretation, self-correction	Hypothetical-deductive reasoning, self-actualization

*From Valett, Robert E., Developing Cognitive Abilities–Teaching Children to Think. St. Louis: C. V. Mosby, 1978, p. 50.

The value of a taxonomy of cognitive skills is that it provides the teacher with a developmental map of possible teaching objectives. Cognitive objectives and skills can be derived from a careful diagnostic evaluation of the dyslexic child and then translated into appropriate lessons and learning activities.

To illustrate the effects of cognitive development programs on reading comprehension and school achievement we will briefly consider the Milwaukee Project. This longitudinal nine-year study is the most extensive of its kind. Forty retarded mothers living in deprived conditions were identified as having children who were high risk cases for repeating the cycle of retardation, school failure, and welfare dependence. The experimental group of twenty children received special instructional interventions that began when they were three months old and continued to the time of their school entry. Nothing was done with the control group of twenty children other than assessment. Mothers were provided with jobs, parent training, and reading and math instruction, and were shown how to stimulate and support their children's development. Early in the program children were read to, taught to follow books, and encouraged to enjoy story time. Creative expression (puppets, dramatics) which entailed much group interaction and sharing of feelings about pictures and stories, was emphasized. Children were told stories, shared stories, and invented stories before they could actually read them. Other parts of the training program included problem-solving and thinking tasks designed to develop verbal expression and comprehension.

Criterion tests on the Milwaukee Project included the Gesell, Binet, Piaget Scales, language tasks, ITPA, and selected matching-sorting discrimination tasks. When the children were fourteen to eighteen months old, significant superiority in language abilities began to appear in the experimental group. From three to five years old, the average sentence length among the experimental group put them a year ahead of the controls. By school age there was a difference of two years in language sophistication over the control group. Garber (1977) reports that in this project the experimental group gradually increased their intelligence test scores to an average of 120, 30 points above the controls. The experimental group also read earlier and better than their schoolmates and were much more verbally aware and sophisticated. These remarkable gains in comprehension and school achievement held up all through the primary grades until the program officially ended in 1977.

What were some of the other cognitive development strategies used in the Milwaukee Project that significantly influenced performance? The experimental group learned through games and systematic learning activities. They received special lessons in comprehension, vocabulary acquisition, symbolic representations, concept evaluation, classification, reversibility, organization of verbal information, and analysis and synthesis of data. The lessons and materials are described in detail by Heber and others (1972).

Naturally, there are many other successful programs for the development of reading comprehension in learning-disabled children. Some of these emphasize the acquisition of meaning and syntax. A doctoral study by Vogel (1975) confirms earlier findings that dyslexic children with reading comprehension problems are deficient in such syntactic abilities as:

- recognizing melody patterns

- comprehending rules of word order in sentences

- ability to repeat sentences correctly

- recognizing common grammatical forms

- correctly expressing words (voice inflection) in sentences in order to convey meaning

Vogel (1977) stresses the importance of morphological deficiencies (failure to recognize forms or to understand them) in dyslexic children and recommends that remedial programs give priority to this area. Wiig and Semel (1976) give numerous strategies for the remediation of cognitive processing deficiencies. Among these strategies are lessons in semantic units that foster understanding of verbs, pronouns, adjectives, prepositions, antonyms, synonyms, homonyms, multiple-meaning words, verbal analogies, idioms, metaphors, and other linguistic abstractions.

One example of a nongraded approach to developing comprehension is Harnadek's Critical Thinking Program. These multilesson books teach basic skills, such as analogies, similarities and differences, synonyms, and elementary logic. Another example is the Think Language Program. Built on the Guilford model, it is a programmed learning approach using 123 tape-cassette lessons. This approach helps secondary students learn to think in terms of things, qualities, classes, structure, events, and relationships, and therefore to comprehend better what they are reading.

BEHAVIORAL SKILLS

By constructing sentences out of words and phrases they know, dyslexic students acquire a knowledge of sentence structure and some linguistic understanding. Through the experimental manipulation of words (such as substituting words in idioms, metaphors, and proverbs) they begin to connect abstractions with their own experiences. As words and phrases are related and organized into logical sentences and paragraphs, comprehension improves. One authority (Strang 1965) summarizes procedures for teaching this kind of meaningful reading and suggests a number of appealing books.

Other authors such as Brueckner and Bond (1955, p. 172) also stress that the development of comprehension is the major objective of all reading instruction. "The child should at all times be reading for definite purposes which demand an understanding of the material read." According to these authorities, there are five major kinds of reading comprehension:

- retention of information (isolating facts and details)
- organization of information (establishing relationships and sequences, summarizing)
- evaluation (establishing cause and effect, judging content relevance, critical appraisal)
- interpretation (recognizing main ideas, inferences, conclusions)
- appreciation (enjoying, sensing tone and humor)

Almost all of these comprehension skills are now being evaluated through the use of state-mandated reading tests. The reading comprehension section of the California Achievement Test covers the following skills:

- following instructions (definitions, choices, directions)
- reference skills (parts of books, table of contents, graph and map reading, alphabetizing, use of index)
- interpretation of material (topic or central idea, inferences, topic organization, direct facts, sequence of events

All other standardized achievement tests have similar reading comprehension sections. In addition to the use of standardized tests, most school districts and clinics have devised supplemental criterion tasks and objectives that help to determine the level of other basic skills such as listening, picture interpretation, and meaningful punctuation. Diagnostic-prescriptive teachers should analyze test results to isolate those specific deficiencies requiring remediation.

Children with special problems in these comprehension skills should be placed in reading programs in which goals are clearly established and relevant. Developmental language experience approaches using multisensory techniques are usually required for teaching these skills to dyslexic children. Many prescriptive programs use "cloze" techniques for diagnostic and instructional purposes. In the cloze technique, a word is removed from a sentence and the child is asked to supply the missing word. Essentially, cloze is a test of the subject's ability to infer the missing word from the syntactic and semantic structures of the remainder of the sentence (Dale 1972). Considerable research has been done on the cloze technique, and Robinson (1971) has compiled an extensive bibliography of studies.

Among the many commercial publications that develop reading comprehension is the Science Research Associates' **Basic Reading Series,** which attempts to integrate structured linguistics and comprehension. SRA also publishes a **Reading Laboratory Series,** which consists of boxed kits of progressively graded short stories with appropriate study questions and activities. The Reader's Digest **Skill Builder** program consists of boxed short stories that are well illustrated and interesting. The **Skyline Series,** published by McGraw Hill's Webster Division, has been developed for culturally underprivileged children and emphasizes picture stories with characters from minority groups. The Allied Education Council's **Fitzhugh Plus Language Program** includes a number of workbooks using cloze techniques. The **Reading-Thinking Skills** workbooks by Continental Press stress high-level skills such as evaluation, inference, organization, and generalization. All these programs provide a source of lesson ideas and learning activities and can be modified for prescriptive use with dyslexic children.

Real life encounters and problems can sometimes develop reading skills as effectively as books and special reading programs. This is especially important in junior and senior high school. The "Functional Reading Skills Chart" (below) shows how many commonly available reading materials can be used to help students apply and develop their skills.

ACTIVE INVOLVEMENT

Since dyslexic children have neuropsychological processing dysfunctions, lessons that call for manipulation of materials and active movement of their bodies in perceptual-linguistic games help to focus attention, contribute to hemispheric integration, and further cognitive development and comprehension.

FUNCTIONAL READING SKILLS

Preschool years:	Primary years:	Elementary years:
Sensory motor play	Laterality-directionality training	Structural-contextual analysis and interpretation
Auditory-visual discrimination	Visual coordination and tracking	Vocabulary expansion
Rhyming	Auditory-vocal synthesis	Free library selection
Story telling	Word attack skills (grapheme/phoneme correspondence: consonants, vowels, blends, syllabication)	Reference skills
Developmental oral language		Comprehension-thinking skills
Temporal ordering	Meaningful experience stories	
Listening and attending	Auditory-visual memory	
	Sight word experiential vocabulary	

Secondary years:		
Comic strips	Payroll deduction forms	Holiday articles and brochures
Neighborhood signs	Rental agreements	Help wanted ads
Menus	Election ballots	Special catalogs (Sears, Radio Shack)
Store sales	Letters from family and friends	Automobile advertising and brochures
News headlines	Movie titles and schedules	Self-selected books
Greeting cards	Food store advertisements	Tax forms
Community and state maps	Sports headlines and articles	Marriage/living together contracts
Popular magazines	Weather reports	Editorials
Medicine ads and labels	Hobby instructions	
Job applications	Music record labels	
Contraceptive information		
Musical record lyrics		

Cratty studied the use of movement to elicit higher-level cognitive ability among learning-handicapped children. Cratty found that more than one cognitive operation should be built into such active movement tasks and that decision making should be transferred to the children as soon as possible (Cratty 1971a; Cratty and Martin 1971). A child's comprehension and application of phonics and other reading skills improves if he or she is involved in active movement but does not improve with passive tutoring. Cratty (1971b) has devised an active learning program to help improve children's memory, categorization, evaluation, and problem-solving skills. Some of the activities for improving reading comprehension include having children:

- read and act out words (*skip, jump, run*)
- use hopscotch word grids (children jump to a word, then use that word in a story)
- write simple stories that they then enact on the playground or in the gymnasium
- participate in chalkboard writing-relay games
- play "steal-the-word" (a modification of "steal-the-bacon") team games using the words in sentences and stories

Rowen (1963) has written an excellent list of stories, poems, and language-comprehension activities. The list includes ways of having children enact words (*sticky, bumpy, hot, shiver, angry, sleeping*) in stories. Rich and Nedboy (1977) report on a similar program, which involved twelve- to fifteen-year-old students with several years of unsuccessful remedial reading. In a poetry-writing exercise, each student was asked to contribute a line to a poem on the chalkboard. Reading comprehension improved dramatically and "poetry production groups" gave students motivation for participation in yet other language development activities. Wilson (1972) advocates that remedial reading begin with field trips, personal stories, model building, science experiments, newspaper and sports column interpretations, or similar activities that the child can enjoy and comprehend. With severe dyslexics, the use of music therapy—including listening to and interpreting lyrics of popular tunes, singing, and dancing—is frequently helpful. Even sign language may be employed with some children if it helps them to understand words.

Active involvement and movement education programs should not be substituted for the structured prescriptive auditory and visual processing training that dyslexic children may require (Vaille 1975). The development of reading comprehension in dyslexic children is founded on the remediation of basic perceptual-linguistic deficiencies and the acquisition of compensatory skills and abilities. But involving severely reading-disabled children in active games and programs also will be required if reading is to become a meaningful and enjoyable experience.

SUMMARY

Dyslexic children can be helped to improve their reading comprehension. Like other human abilities, reading comprehension develops through instruction and practice.

Severely disabled children must be motivated to develop a positive anticipatory set or readiness to participate in reading. Language development activities help to further meaning and comprehension.

There are many cognitive skills that contribute to the development of reading comprehension. Many of these skills and abilities have been summarized in various taxonomies that can be useful to the special educator. Mental abilities and cognitive operations can be developed through prescriptive instruction.

Many of the specific behavioral skills required for comprehending reading material are measured by standardized achievement and criterion tests. Items from these instruments should be used as a possible source of remedial tasks and objectives. Most dyslexic children require remedial training in semantic relationships and in meaningful interpretation of words and phrases.

Reading comprehension can be furthered through active involvement and multisensory learning activities. For dyslexic children, such involvement serves to integrate neuropsychological processing skills and contributes to hemispheric organization and the better understanding of abstract concepts.

Five comprehension lessons follow.

Objective: to understand, interpret, and reenact a short story

Materials: worksheet, story props, crayons, paper

Directions: Read this story and complete the learning activities that follow. Pay special attention to the words that are underlined.

Unidentified Flying Object

Tom woke up in bed. His radio and television set were going on and off. Then
he noticed the minute and hour hands on his electric clock spinning around
very fast. Suddenly a strange red light shone through the window and Tom
heard a loud noise outside. It sounded something like a jet.

   He quickly got out of bed and looked out at the empty lot next to his home.
A huge blue saucerlike object was slowly landing on the grass. A strange kind
of person seemed to be waving to him from a hole in the side of the unusual
aircraft. Then very weird things began to happen.

1. What happened to Tom's radio and television set?
2. What color was the light that shone through the window?
3. Describe what was happening outside the house.
4. Color a picture of the UFO using the description given in the story.
5. What do you think might happen next?
6. Discuss an ending to this story with another student. Together write a con-
   cluding paragraph or two.

Evaluations:

Task	+	+ /-	-	Comments
1				
2				
3				
4				
5				
6				

Variations: Compile story endings from other pupils. Dramatize the stories. Tape-record
and write original UFO stories and illustrate them with drawings, paintings, and
pictures from newspapers and magazines.

Objective: to remember, sing, enact, and interpret "fun songs" and lyrics

Materials: song sheets, records or cassette tapes, earphone and tape recorder

Directions:

1. Here is the song sheet with the words to "Old MacDonald Had a Farm":

   > Old MacDonald had a farm, e i, e i, oh!
   >
   > And on his farm he had some ducks, e i, e i, oh!
   >
   > With a quack, quack here and a quack, quack there
   >
   > here a quack, there a quack, everywhere quack, quack
   >
   > Old MacDonald had a farm, e i, e i, oh!
   >
   > **Repeat and add pigs (oink, oink), chicks (cluck, cluck), and others.**

   First, let us read the words to the song together. Put your finger under each word as we read it.

2. Now we will listen to this tape recording of the song with music. Listen to the words and music and try to feel the rhythm. Follow the words with your finger as you hear them.

3. This time we will all sing the song together but when we get to the animal sounds we will stand up and sing "quack, quack" and "oink, oink" loud and clear.

4. Put this earphone on your right ear and listen to the taped song by yourself. Without my helping you, follow the words with your fingers. You may sing along with the music if you wish.

5. Sing the song for me without listening to the music or looking at the song sheet.

6. Now look at the song sheet again and

   a. draw a circle around the name of the farmer wherever you see it;

   b. draw a picture of the animals in the song and write or print their names below the picture;

   c. underline the sounds that **one** of the animals makes.

Evaluation: Give a plus mark for each of the above directions followed. Note special errors in auditory-vocal memory and rhythm. Add other animals and comprehension questions and activities.

Variations: Develop more complex auditory-vocal memory and reading comprehension using appropriate nursery rhymes, folk songs, camp songs, and student-selected popular music and lyrics.

Objective: to increase vocabulary, understanding, and word use based on experience

Materials: worksheet

Directions: Here are some words and pictures of things that you used when you dictated your Christmas story into the tape recorder.

apple   pop   cake

candy   bread   cookies

1. Look at each word and picture. Use that word in a sentence and then draw a circle around the word.

2. Point to each word and tell me how it is like the other words. How is it different?

3. Read these words: cake   bread   cookies
   Use each of these words in a sentence. Tell me what these words have in common–in what way are they similar or alike?

4. Draw lines between the words that go together and explain why they go together:

   apple   coke

   bread   chocolate

   pop   bake

   candy   red

5. Draw a line from each word that is underlined to the one word below that "goes best" with it. Tell me why you picked that word.

   <u>apple</u>   <u>candy</u>   <u>cookies</u>   <u>cake</u>

   foot–fruit–fly   shoes–sweet–sour   nuts–nest–night   bake–bird–bear

6. Write a short paragraph using three of the words underlined above.

Evaluation: Number correct _____

                    Kinds of errors _____

Variations: Have students sort and classify the basic Dolch words and words from a basal reader. Let the student eat part of an apple, cookie, or cake, after successful completion of tasks using that word.

Objective: to relate words to one another and interpret their meanings

Materials: worksheet, picture cards

Directions:
1. **Compound words:** Here is a picture of a cow with the word below it. Here is a picture of a boy with the word printed on it. If we put them together we can make up a new word **cowboy**. Here are some other pictures. Put as many of them together as you can to make up a new word, then draw lines between the words below to show the new word:

hand	time	door	pen	arm	man
bed	boat	basket	shoe	pan	pole
cow	bag	horse	bell	flag	chair
sail	boy	pig	ball	mail	cake

2. **Descriptive words:** Draw a line under the word that best describes the first word in the line.

ice:	tall	cold	warm	rich
knife:	dark	blue	sharp	wet
elephant:	huge	hard	not	hit
mountain:	sad	cheap	wise	high
night:	light	green	dark	wide

3. **Words that are out of place:** Cross out the word that does not belong with the others:

- cat   dog   robin   horse
- cup   coat   dish   fork
- nose   ear   house   eye
- boy   Wednesday   Friday   Sunday
- water   tea   milk   bread

continued

4. **Idioms and metaphors:** Read these sentences and tell me what they mean.

- Betty is as busy as a beaver.
- Mark caught a cold.
- Strike while the iron is hot.
- After he won the game he was as pleased as punch.

5. **Inconsistencies and absurdities:** Read these sentences and then change some of the words so that the sentence makes sense.

- George drank the hot dog.
- He took the horse to his garage for repairs.
- Sally hit the football with her racket.
- Yesterday, Joe got burned in the hot rain.
- North is to South as East is to North.
- Tomorrow I will talk with Abraham Lincoln in the White House.
- Man is to woman as boy is to dog.

Evaluation:

Task	Number correct	Kinds of errors
1		
2		
3		
4		
5		

Variations: Make tasks more difficult. Place a "daily proverb" on the bulletin board for discussion. Have students write or bring in their own special word problems.

Objective: to be able to "cloze" sentences using the proper word or words to convey meaning.

Materials: worksheet

Directions: Read the following sentences and fill in the missing words:

1. Jane got a new ten-speed _____ for her birthday.

2. A _____ is a very tall, long-necked animal with spots on its skin.

3. Earth is _____ of the nine planets.

4. The _____ of the United States is Washington, D.C.

5. Most fish can't _____ out of water.

6. I pledge _____ to the flag of the United _____ of America.

7. McDonald's restaurants _____ hamburgers and other fast foods.

8. Dan's dog liked to _____ after squirrels. The squirrels always got away by _____ trees.

9. May saw some bears and lions in the _____. She also saw a huge _____ with a long trunk and thick legs. People were throwing peanuts to the _____ who were swinging in their cages.

10. Most planes cannot fly faster than the _____ of sound, _____ a modern jet can.

Evaluation: Number correct _____

Kinds of errors _____

Variations: Have students block out words in old books, magazines, or newspapers to give to one another.

DISCUSSION QUESTIONS AND ACTIVITIES

1. Define *syntax* and discuss its importance.

2. Administer a reading comprehension test to a dyslexic child and analyze the results.

3. Evaluate a dyslexic pupil and discuss what might motivate that child to develop a more positive "set" for reading.

4. Write a critique of one model of cognitive abilities (Piaget, Guilford, Bloom, and others).

5. Select two teaching skills from the "Cognitive Skills Instructional Taxonomy" (Table 6) for use with a dyslexic child you have evaluated.

6. Why do you think the Milwaukee Project was successful in developing reading comprehension among the children who participated?

7. Demonstrate one of the commercial programs mentioned in this chapter.

8. Review and report on the results of the state-required reading comprehension section of the test used in one of the local grade schools. What skills did students seem to have most difficulty with? What are some of the implications of these test results?

9. Design, teach, and evaluate a reading comprehension lesson for a dyslexic child using active involvement learning tasks.

Through the use of these educational methods and principles, an
inferior mentality would be able to
grow and develop.

Maria Montessori

CHAPTER TWELVE

Reading Resource Materials

The modern special educator is fortunate to have a wide variety of
instructional materials and programs to choose from. These include
many good remedial reading materials that can be adapted for supplemental use with dyslexic children. This chapter lists some reading
resource materials currently in use in many special education and
clinical programs. A brief description of each item is presented, but
readers should consult the appendix for publishers' addresses and cor-
respond with them for detailed information.

TESTS AND EVALUATION INSTRUMENTS

Included are several tests and clinical instruments useful in diagnostic
and teaching programs.

The Halstead-Reitan Neuropsychological Test Battery. Two major approaches to the evaluation of neuropsychological dysfunction are
currently used by psychologists in clinical programs. One of these is
qualitative assessment as developed by Luria and as described by
Christensen (1975). The other is the quantitative psychometric test
originally developed by Halstead (1947) and subsequently refined by

Reitan and Davidson (1974). Special educators working with dyslexic children should be aware that the Halstead-Reitan battery, published by Ralph Reitan Neuropsychological Laboratory, consists of the following subtests:

- a category test (abstract ability)
- a tactual performance test (blindfolded manipulated memory)
- the Seashore Rhythm test (discriminating musical beats)
- a speech-sounds perception test (discriminating between similar-sounding consonants)
- a finger tapping test (coordination and sensory integration)

In addition to the above, psychologists will add some of the following: the Trail-Making (visual-motor tracing) Test; the Halstead Aphasia Screening Test; finger agnosia, skin writing, and sensory extinction tasks; the Wechsler Intelligence Scale; and the Minnesota Multiphasic Personality Inventory.

Laboratory Instruments. Some clinical equipment and instruments useful with dyslexic children and available through the Lafayette Instrument Company are listed below:

- Electro-Tach (A special tachistoscopic machine for individual use)
- various standard tachistoscopes
- audiometers
- electric counters and timers
- mazes
- rotary pursuit apparatus
- cutaneous sensitivity kits
- blindfold goggles
- vibrometers
- metronomes
- visual stimulators
- reaction speed timers
- psychogalvanometers
- portable EEG units
- delayed feedback machines

The Biofeedback Research Institute markets an electromyograph, galvanic skin response apparatus, digital integrator, EEG feedback device, and a highly effective digital thermometer useful in self-control programs.

SOBAR Criterion Tests.   These criterion reading objectives were developed at UCLA through a National Institute of Education project. SOBAR stands for the **S**ystem for **O**bjective-**B**ased **A**ssessment of **R**eading. Objectives cover letter recognition, phonic analysis, structural analysis, vocabulary, comprehension, and study skills. There are 162 objectives for grades K–2, and 140 objectives for grades 3–9.

TABLE 7.   Dolch Basic 220 Words

These words are said to constitute 75 percent of all words used in first-grade reading and 65 percent of all other primary books.

Easier Half

Should be fixed as sight words by the end of first grade. These are also known as the Popper Words, Group I

a	away	can	find	good	his	like	old	run	that	we
after	be	carry	five	green	I	little	on	said	the	went
all	big	cold	fly	had	if	look	one	saw	this	what
am	black	come	for	has	in	make	out	see	three	who
an	blue	did	from	have	into	may	over	she	to	will
and	brown	do	funny	he	is	me	play	so	too	with
are	but	don't	get	help	it	my	put	some	two	yellow
around	by	down	give	her	its	no	ran	soon	under	yes
as	call	eat	go	here	jump	not	red	stop	up	you
at	came	fast	going	him	know	of	ride	ten	was	your

Harder Half

Should be fixed by the end of second grade. These are also known as the Popper Words, Group II

about	better	drink	goes	laugh	never	pick	show	their	try	were
again	both	eight	got	let	new	please	sing	them	upon	when
always	bring	every	grow	light	now	pretty	sit	then	us	where
any	buy	fall	hold	live	off	pull	six	there	use	which
ask	clean	far	hot	long	once	read	sleep	these	very	white
ate	could	first	how	made	only	right	small	they	walk	why
because	cut	found	hurt	many	open	round	start	think	want	wish
been	does	four	just	much	or	say	take	those	warm	work
before	done	full	keep	must	our	seven	tell	today	wash	would
best	draw	gave	kind	myself	own	shall	thank	together	well	write

Mastery tests are available for all skills. The entire program is published by Science Research Associates.

Dolch Words.   The practical work of Edward Dolch (1960) has long been used by special educators. His list of 220 basic words (Table 7) and the list of common nouns (Table 8) should be used as criterion test words with dyslexic children. A series of basic word games, kits, and workbooks are available from Garrard Publishing Company (and most teacher supply houses) and should be used in all developmental-remedial reading programs.

The Verbal Opposites Test.   Table 9 is an adaptation of verbal opposites from the Detroit Tests of Learning Aptitude by Baker and Lea-

TABLE 8.   Picture Words–The 95 Commonest Nouns (Dolch)

airplane	children	hand	rabbit
apple	coat	hat	rain
baby	corn	head	ring
back	cow	hen	road
ball	dog	hill	school
barn	doll	horse	sheep
basket	door	house	shoe
bear	dress	kitten	snow
bed	duck	leg	squirrel
bell	ear	letter	stick
bird	eggs	man	store
birthday	elephant	men	street
boat	eye	milk	sun
book	face	money	table
box	farm	monkey	tail
boy	father	mother	toys
bread	feet	nest	train
bus	fire	nose	tree
cake	fish	paper	wagon
cap	flower	party	watch
car	garden	picture	water
cat	girl	pig	window
chair	grass	pony	wood
chicken	hair	puppy	

land. The test is very helpful in determining a child's potential reading ability, since it samples his or her comprehension of words in several different ways.

The teacher first says to the child, "If I say the word *boy* to you,

TABLE 9. The Verbal Opposites Test (Valett Adaptation)

Stimulus	Correct Response	M.A. (G.P.)	Stimulus	Correct Response	M.A. (G.P.)
1. boy	girl		31. narrow	wide	9-3
2. front	back		32. false	true	9-6 (4-3)
3. up	down		33. love	hate	9-6
4. brother	sister		34. remember	forget	9-9 (4.5)
5. wet	dry	5-6	35. pretty	ugly	10-O
6. dirty	clean	5-9	36. stale	fresh	10-O (4.7)
7. young	old	5-9	37. blonde	brunette	10-3
8. hot	cold	6-O	38. absent	present, here	10-3 (4.9)
9. dead	alive	6-O	39. same	different	10-6
10. crooked	straight	6-3 (1.O)	40. raw	cooked	10-6 (5.1
11. early	late	6-6 (1.2)	41. cruel	kind	10-9
12. sour	sweet	6-6 (1.4)	42. after	before	10-9 (5.4)
13. shut	open	6-9 (1.6)	43. sharp	dull	11-O (5.6)
14. empty	full	7-O (1.8)	44. evening	morning	11-3 (5.9)
15. late	early	7-O	45. friend	enemy	11-6 (6.1)
16. tight	loose	7-3 (2.O)	46. multiply	divide	11-9 (6.4)
17. lost	found	7-6	47. wild	tame	12-O (6.6)
18. north	south	7-8 (2.3)	48. public	private	12-3 (6.9)
19. sick	well	7-9 (2.5)	49. dangerous	safe	12-6 (7.1)
20. off	on	7-9	50. victory	defeat	12-9 (7.3)
21. black	white	8-O (2.8)	51. begin	end, stop	13-O (7.6)
22. heavy	light	8-3	52. deep	shallow	13-3 (7.9)
23. near	far	8-3 (3.O)	53. difficult	easy	13-6 (8.1)
24. smooth	rough	8-6	54. lengthen	shorten	13-9 (8.4)
25. asleep	awake	8-6 (3.3)	55. costly	cheap	14-O (8.6)
26. come	go	8-9 (3.5)	56. succeed	fail	14-3 (8.8)
27. add	subtract	8-9	57. imprisoned	free	14-6 (9.O)
28. laugh	cry	9-O (3.7)	58. entrance	exit	14-9 (9.2)
29. daughter	son	9-O	59. falsehood	truth	15-O (9.5)
30. strong	weak	9-3 (4.O)	60. lend	borrow	15-3 (9.8)

what word means just the opposite? Yes, *girl* is the opposite of *boy*."
Then the teacher pronounces each word and waits for the child's verbal response. When a child misses a word, the teacher writes down the
incorrect answer for later consideration. Occasionally one should ask
the child to use the antonym in a sentence to be sure he or she knows
what it means. One continues the test until the subject has made five
consecutive errors. Note that Table 9 gives mental age (M.A.) and
approximate grade placement score (G.P.), which is in parentheses
and derived from the tables of Thomas and Cresimbeni (1966).

In a second testing, the child *reads* the stimulus word with the correct responses covered, then gives the antonym. The test can be given a
third time by having the child read the stimulus word and *write* the opposite word, or the stimulus word can be read by the teacher while the
student writes the response. Carefully note the discrepancy in all scores
and evaluate all responses in terms of their implication for prescriptive
instruction.

PROGRAMMED LEARNING EQUIPMENT

Included are programs ranging from a series of question cards to
teaching machines.

Tutorgram.   This teaching aid from the Enrichment Reading Corporation of America uses programmed cards to teach language and
other concepts. The cards are in color with pictured multiple-choice
responses. When the child marks the right answer he or she is reinforced with a light and buzzer.

Friendly Tutor.   Creative Teaching Associates makes this plastic
and wood board that covers electric circuits operating on a single flashlight battery. There are fourteen different program sets (each with sixteen cards of ten problems), including visual discrimination, auditory
discrimination, consonants, blends, digraphs, vowels, compound
words, antonyms, synonyms, homonyms, prefixes, and suffixes.

EP Basic Reading Program.   Educational Projections Company
manufactures this self-instructional system. The Multiple-choice Programmed Viewer allows a student to study the frame, select an answer,
and be rewarded by a green light and buzzer if the answer is right.
After making a correct choice, the student moves on to the next frame.

If the answer is wrong, the student studies the frame again and makes another selection. There are 440 developmental-sequential lessons on filmstrips and cassettes, beginning with reading-readiness skills and proceeding through fifth-grade level.

REC Talking Page. The "Talking Page," by Response Environments Corporation, is a small portable machine combining textbook reading with an audio-visual desk-top learning system. The program consists of a series of books and recorded discs usually used with earphones by individual students. Materials are story-based, well illustrated, and highly motivating for young children. Skill sequences include auditory discrimination, visual discrimination, and language growth (vocabulary, classification, comprehension, prepositional relationships).

ETA Electronic Reading System. This unit by Educational Teaching Aids includes a scanning table on which any printed reading material may be placed for magnification (six to thirty times normal). The scanner moves laterally and from front to back and the readout is on a fourteen-inch television monitor. This unit provides individually controlled magnification and self-pacing for persons with visual problems.

DEVELOPMENTAL READINESS PROGRAMS

The list includes programs for very young children, preschool and kindergarten children, and older children with learning disabilities.

RADEA. The goal of this program by Melton Book Company is to increase adaptive behaviors in severely handicapped children from birth to seven years old. Several hundred visual perception, auditory perception, perceptual motor, oral language, and functional living skills are grouped in four levels. Lessons are provided on color-coded task cards for use in sequential instruction. The program also includes screening tests, cassettes, picture cards, progress charts, and profiles.

Learning Language at Home. In this kit by the Council for Exceptional Children there are individual lesson plans for parents and teachers of three- to five-year-old children. A total of two thousand sequenced lesson cards with one thousand manipulative learning activities are provided. Emphasis is on cognitive and intellectual develop-ment in four skill areas: learning to do, learning to look, learning to listen, and learning to tell.

Santa Clara Plus.   Richard L. Zweig Associates, Inc. put out this developmental program for preschool-kindergarten children. There are 242 readiness activity cards that provide sequential lessons in motor coordination, visual-motor performance, visual perception, visual memory, auditory perception, auditory memory, language develop-ment, and conceptual development.

The Perceptual Skills Curriculum.   The Walker Educational Book Corporation publishes this preschool, grade 1, and special edu-cation program of tests and correlated activities in basic reading, writing, arithmetic, and spelling. The curriculum includes 133 se-quenced educational objectives paired with criterion-referenced tests and hundreds of learning activities. The four programs cover visual-motor skills, auditory-motor skills, and general motor skills and intro-duce letters and numerals. Individual worksheets are correlated with sensory-motor manipulative activities.

Perceive and Respond Auditory Program.   This special auditory training program was designed by the Modern Education Corporation for use by both special educators and regular classroom teachers. Vol-ume 1 covers environmental sounds with nine cassette tapes and self-correcting answer sheets. Volume 2 covers auditory discrimination of consonants, words, rhythm, phrases, and blends with twelve tapes. Volume 3 has five taped lessons on auditory sequential memory skills.

Peace, Harmony, and Awareness Self-Management Tapes.   This relaxation program by Melton Book Company is for use with learning-disabled hyperactive children. The six cassette tapes are designed for use with preschool to intermediate age children and can be used in reg-ular classrooms, resource rooms, clinics, or special classes. Children are taught to reduce muscle tension, to use their imaginations in dealing more effectively with stressful situations, and to relax in several differ-ent ways.

Edmark Reading Program.   Edmark Associates designed this pro-gram for use with the severely handicapped. It is a developmental reading program that uses sequential teaching frames and provides behavioral feedback. Essentially, this is a programmed sight-word vocabulary that is taught through short lessons requiring the student to point to and read words and phrases. Lessons are grouped into five major sequences: prereading, word recognition, direction book, picture/ phrase matching, and storybook reading.

PIPER. These "**P**rescriptive **I**nstructional **P**rograms for **E**ducational **R**eadiness" by Reader's Digest Services, Inc. develop 157 measurable competencies in the five skill areas of gross-motor control ("willows"), visual-motor processes ("windows"), auditory processes ("waves"), language skills ("whispers"), and reasoning abilities ("wonders"). Materials are packaged in kits and include activity guides, record cards, and duplicating lesson master worksheets. For example, "Wonders: Reasoning Abilities" has lessons and activities in categorization, classification, seriation, generalization, and comparisons; in proposing alternatives, making inferences, and analyzing facts; and in inductive and deductive reasoning.

PRIMARY READING MATERIALS

Varied reading programs from phonics to multisensory methods are included here.

Developing Reading Skills. This filmstrip series by Educational Enrichment Materials accompanies basal readers. Four sets of strips cover word perception, vowel sounds, consonants b to m, and consonants n to z. Each set includes six color filmstrips with accompanying records or cassettes, student workbooks, and a teacher's guide. Since the filmstrips are full of humor, these lessons are enjoyable for young children.

Fun with Phonics. Highlights for Children, Inc. publishes this series of special "handbooks," useful as supplemental material. This phonics booklet is recommended for parents who work with their child at home.

The Johnny Right-to-Read Program. Here is a unique multisensory program by Academic Therapy Publications. It develops reading skills and writing expression in disabled children and adults. The program fosters recognition and use of symbol-sound association, mastery of blends, and success in long and short vowel perception and discrimination. Compensatory procedures are also cultivated to help overcome deficiencies. Constant multisensory feedback is provided along with the use of behavior modification techniques.

Syntax One.   These materials were designed by Communication Skill Builders, Inc. for the child with syntactic skills lagging one to five years behind other language-related skills. They consist of six double-sided syntax wheels depicting the sentence construction to be taught. Charts, workbooks, and a teacher's manual are included in the kit.

Developmental Syntax Program.   Learning Concepts publishes this series of eight programs for correcting expressive syntax disorders in children three to ten years old. The programs are based on the most common syntactical errors recorded in young children and teach adjectives, personal pronouns, possessive pronouns, the verbs *is* and *are,* the verbs *has* and *have,* plurality, and the past tense of regular and irregular verbs.

The Pelican Series.   Utilizing a developmental approach, this program by Allyn and Bacon, Inc. combines critical skills in word attack, phonics, comprehension, and recognition of linguistic spelling patterns with spelling and writing activities. This series of four books was developed by special educators for use with learning-handicapped children and prepares children for transition to basal readers. Materials include books, duplicating masters, and teacher's manuals.

Tales of Fantasy and Music and **Fables of Aesop.**   Prentice-Hall Media publish these imaginative stories that encourage children to listen thoughtfully, observe carefully, speak effectively, and write creatively. Six colorful filmstrips have specially composed music on cassettes or records. The material from Aesop is especially designed to motivate poor readers, is captioned to match the narration, and gives the child practice in new words and unfamiliar sentence structure.

Learning with Laughter.   This program by Prentice-Hall Media uses filmstrips, cassettes, charts, picture cards, and puppets to teach consonants, blends, vowels, inflectional endings, and frequently used words. Colorful cartoon characters in the filmstrips engage children in marching tunes, limericks, songs, games, and manipulative learning activities. This is a highly motivating program for young children with basic reading problems.

Dr. Seuss Beginning Readers.   Random House has had great success with this highly appealing series of beginning readers that introduce controlled vocabulary words systematically yet in creative and imaginative ways. Many books in this series, such as *The Cat in the Hat, Hop on Pop, Fox in Socks, Dr. Seuss ABC's, Cat in the Hat Comes Back,* and *Green Eggs and Ham* have become classics in remedial reading programs.

ELEMENTARY READING MATERIALS

More advanced reading programs are included under this heading.

First Thinking Box I, and **Thinking Skills Development Program II.**   This program by Benefic Press contains three levels of lesson material: Level one—observing, comparing, classifying, imagining; Level two—hypothesizing, criticizing, looking for assumptions, collecting and organizing data; Level three—summarizing, coding, interpreting, problem solving.

Box I covers grades 3–5. Box II is for use with grades 6–9. Each box contains twelve filmstrips, cassettes, skill development cards, thinking cards, reference books, record sheets, and a teacher's guide.

BFA Comprehension Skill Laboratory.   This laboratory kit by BFA Educational Media provides activities in the following four major skill areas:

- information skills
  recalling facts and details
  paraphrasing

- organization skills
  determining sequence
  following directions
  classifying

- generalization skills
  titling
  identifying main ideas
  summarizing

- evaluation skills
    - making inferences
    - drawing conclusions
    - predicting outcomes
    - judging relevance and significance
    - comparing and contrasting
    - recognizing emotional attitudes
    - forming sensory images
    - characterizing

Materials consist of 232 color-coded instructional cards, story cards, diagnostic-placement tests, answer sheets, and review activities. Eight different laboratory kits are available on developmental readability or classroom levels.

LSI Reading Skills Development. Learning Skills, Inc. packages six kits of independent reading activities that teach phonics, word structure, vocabulary, comprehension, and research and study skills. Kits contain skill activity cards, answer sheets, progress charts, and manuals. Student self-recording of scores for each completed activity is an important part of this program.

SRA Corrective Reading Program. This program by Science Research Associates is for students in grades 4–12 who have not yet mastered decoding skills. Instruction is presented in basic word-attack skills, decoding strategies, skill applications, thinking, and comprehension. Highly structured stories with frequent word repetition are presented. The program uses short sentences, constant feedback, and a behavior modification point system that provides constant positive reinforcement. Materials include placement test, stories, work sheets, score and record forms, and manuals.

The NFL Reading Kit. This high-interest, easy-reading kit by Bowmar Publishing Corporation combines the excitement of football with the development of basic reading skills. The reading level of this material is from 2.0 to 4.25; it is thus useful for older students who have extreme reading difficulties. Fifty football stories are arranged into five reading levels. Comprehension check sheets are used with each story. When a student completes a portion of the kit satisfactorily, he is awarded an "NFL reading improvement certificate."

SECONDARY AND ADULT MATERIALS

Programs for persons beyond the early school years are included below.

Pacemaker Bestellers.   This collection by Fearon Pitman Publishers, Inc. features thirty low-reading-level, high-interest paperback books that entice reluctant readers. These books use the Pacemaker Core Vocabulary of 1,021 words that are read with 95 percent accuracy by older students reading at the third-grade level. Contemporary themes and high adventure plots with good illustrations make these books very useful.

The Productive Thinking Program.   Charles E. Merrill Publishing Company produces this course in learning to think. It develops inquiry skills and stresses problem-solving techniques used in language arts, reading, and other subjects. Each of the five programs contains fifteen lessons, duplicating masters, "thinking guides," record charts, and a teacher's guide.

Language Structure Simplified.   Available through Educational Activities, Inc., this series of five developmental kits presents pictures and printed words to teach basic language formulation and syntax. Skills taught are present-tense action sentences, prepositions, plurals, pronoun usage, future-present-past tense sentences, and comparative adjectives. Two of the kits are especially designed for adults or older students using the same format but more appropriate pictures and visual aids.

Handtalk.   This primer of finger spelling and sign language is published by Childcraft Educational Corporation. The lessons introduce the finger-spelling alphabet, encourage self-expression, and reinforce alphabet-reading-spelling skills. Lessons are presented in photographs and wall charts. Although useful at all levels, this approach may be especially helpful for older students with auditory-receptive and expressive handicaps who require compensatory training.

Innerchange.   This new curriculum, by Pennant Educational Materials, is intended for junior and senior high school students with objectives in the *affective* domain. Over forty instructional units on such themes as communication, creativity, life and death, careers, sex roles, and justice involve readers in high-interest reading tasks and activities. This company distributes a "Wishbook" catalog for teachers, which lists books, duplicator lessons, and reading materials for humanizing the learning experience.

Galaxy 5 Series.   Published by Fearon Pitman Publishers, Inc., this series of six short science fiction novels has been designed for junior and senior high school students and adults reading at the third-grade level. These high-interest books about space travel focus on adult characters in suspenseful and imaginative adventures. Also available are DramaTape™ cassettes that dramatize the opening chapters of each book. The cassettes feature voices of professional actors, musical background, and sound effects. The tapes allow students to listen as they read the first two chapters of each book and motivate them to continue reading to find out how each story ends.

Specter Series.   Also by Fearon Pitman Publishers, Inc., this collection of eight low-reading level, high-interest novels motivates junior and senior high school students and adults to read. These are out-of-the-ordinary ghost stories. The themes of mystery and occult and psychic phenomena are treated in nontraditional ways. Repeated word usage in description and simple sentence construction help develop word recognition and comprehension skills. The books have a 2.6 grade reading level.

SUMMARY   The list of selected reading resource materials in this chapter gives an idea of the range of instructional aids currently in use.

Supplemental tests and evaluations can suggest additional prescriptive teaching possibilities. Standardized tests, clinical evaluation, and criterion objectives and inventories all contribute information to the special educator. The verbal-opposites test is an example of an instrument that is helpful in establishing a child's comprehension and potential for reading.

Programmed learning equipment is gaining acceptance in remedial programs and clinics. Teaching machines and programs vary in size and cost. Most schools and clinics could benefit by using programmed learning machines and lessons to supplement and reinforce instruction.

Severe reading disabilities can be prevented partially through the adoption by the school of a well-organized developmental readiness program. These programs are ungraded and allow children to grow and learn at their own rates through the stimulation of appropriate lessons and activities. Almost all dyslexic children require early identification and placement in a program that permits them to make continuous progress yet allows for prescriptive remedial training.

Of course, schools and remedial reading clinics must also provide a variety of reading materials: remedial kits and programs to supplement basal readers and library books; carefully selected, highly attractive contemporary materials on all reading levels from preschool through high school; and special materials on all levels to help dyslexic children improve their thinking and comprehension skills.

DISCUSSION QUESTIONS AND ACTIVITIES

1. Discuss what kinds of neuropsychological tests have been used by consulting psychologists in work with dyslexic children. How can these test results be used by special educators?

2. Demonstrate the use of the tachistoscope in developmental-remedial reading.

3. Select and discuss a list of criterion objectives for reading.

4. Devise a tape-recorded lesson using some of the Dolch words.

5. Administer the verbal-opposites test to a dyslexic child. Report the discrepancy between the child's verbal response, oral reading response, and written response. Compare these results with other test information and discuss the child's potential for learning to read.

6. Go to an instructional media resource center, select a specific programmed learning machine and lesson, and describe how it might be used with dyslexic children.

7. Demonstrate one of the developmental readiness programs described in this chapter. How might it possibly help to *prevent* severe reading disorders?

8. Write a critique of a primary reading program that is used with reading-disabled children.

9. Visit a local school to observe the remedial reading books and materials in use. Describe these to your discussion group.

10. Make a list of high-interest, low-reading-level materials (books, magazines, contemporary musical lyrics, and so forth) that might be used to motivate older dyslexic pupils.

I view education as the most
important subject which we,
as a people, can be engaged in.
                        Abraham Lincoln

CHAPTER THIRTEEN

School
and Clinical Organization

In this chapter, we will consider some aspects of school and clinic organization that influence the behavior of dyslexic children. Several proposals will be made for designing more effective organizational systems and involving teachers and parents in bringing these about.

MATURATIONAL DIFFERENCES IN CHILDREN

Dyslexic children require school placement at their own developmental achievement levels and should not be placed arbitrarily in grades according to chronological age.

But there is another part of this school placement problem that requires some elaboration: maturational differences among non-dyslexic boys and girls, and their effect upon school performance. Most school systems have preferred to deny or ignore basic maturational and achievement differences between the sexes, but sex-maturational differences should affect how the early school years are organized. Here are some of the more important behavioral differences that have been found to exist between males and females.

One of the more popular summaries of these differences is by Rader (1977). Boys are frailer and more vulnerable to stress and sickness than girls, a vulnerability that persists throughout life and makes for the earlier death of males. Boys have higher metabolic rates than girls and are therefore more active and find it harder to sit still. Their greater respiration rates, lung capacities, and muscle strength make them less tolerant of idleness and boredom. However, boys' small hand muscles develop sixteen months later than girls'. A boy's wrist-movement control also develops later and his hands tire more quickly in writing and drawing activities. More boys than girls are brain-injured and mentally retarded. The incidence of allergic reactions or genetic predisposition to allergic reactions is nine times higher in boys than girls (Feingold 1973). Smith (1976) reports that boys are more likely to have genetically based hyperactive predispositions than girls (four to one) and a higher incidence of medical problems such as hypoglycemia, diabetes, and enzyme malfunctions.

Girls begin to develop cognitive skills much more quickly than boys. They speak earlier, have larger vocabularies, and use longer and more complex sentences. These differences produce a more rapid rate of learning in girls, which results in higher intelligence test and achievement test scores. Block and Dworkin (1976) remind us that on the first Stanford-Binet intelligence tests, girls' scores were 2 to 4 percent higher than boys' *at every age level*. However, in subsequent revision of this test and many others, the items were manipulated to bring about equal average scores for males and females. David Wechsler reports that females do better on vocabulary items (while males do better on individual arithmetic tests) and that they have higher mean intelligence test scores at almost every age level, which fact he interpreted as "demonstrating the measurable superiority of women over men so far as general intelligence is concerned" (Wechsler 1944, p. 107).

Numerous studies show the superiority of girls in academic learning during the kindergarten-primary years, when they significantly outperform boys in all areas (Kagan 1964). Among those with reading problems, the ratio of boys to girls ranges from 3:1 to 6:1, depending upon age and level. On readiness and achievement tests in grades 1 and 2, girls make significantly higher scores in visual and auditory discrimination, general reading ability, spelling, language, and arithmetic (Dykstra and Tinney 1969). Girls begin to achieve better than boys in kindergarten as evidenced by higher performance in specific readiness skills (Stanchfield 1971). Extensive reading test results show that girls learn to read earlier than boys (Anderson, Hughes, and Dixon 1956) and that they do better on intersensory symbolic and perceptual functions and on visual-motor tasks (Hirst 1969). By the end of the first grade girls are outperforming boys in reading (Konski 1951), and this superiority continues or slowly increases from the lower to the higher grades (Samuels 1943, Hughes 1953, Gates 1961, Jastak and Jastak 1976).

These differences also appear in studies of special groups. For example, Negro boys perform relatively worse in school than Negro girls; in fact, differences in performance are much greater than in the white population. Furthermore, "it is noteworthy that these sex differences in achievement are observed among southern as well as northern Negroes and are present at every socioeconomic level and tend to increase with age" (Bronfenbrenner 1967, p. 913). Studies of over sixteen thousand hearing-impaired children show that boys consistently scored below girls on tests of paragraph meaning on the Stanford Achievement Tests (Gentile 1973).

However, adolescent boys begin to show superiority on tests of spatial abilities, mechanical reasoning, science, and mathematics. Boys also become more questioning than girls. Girls continue to score better in language areas and are much more imitative of adults. Recent studies by Buffery (1976) show that adult males do better on spatial skills whereas women do better on verbal tests.

There are other indications of more neuropsychological dysfunctions in boys than girls. In a study of growth patterns in children from birth to five years of age, Arnold Gesell (1940) and his colleagues discovered that girls matured more quickly in such fine motor tasks as drawing a man, drawing a circle, and dressing themselves. Most dyslexic children are boys with laterality or mixed dominance problems. We have stated that right-handedness is usually the result of left-hemispheric dominance. Left-handedness, however, is the result of *mixed* cerebral dominance, where neither the right nor left hemisphere has complete control of the body. During the early developmental years, children achieving well academically and socially reflect normal cerebral maturation as evidenced by drawing circles in a counter-clockwise direction with either hand. Left-handed dyslexic children show mixed left-circling and right-circling behavior (called *torque*) that is interpreted by Blau (1977) as an external manifestation of a neural integrative defect in the corpus callosum. The corpus callosum is a rather large connecting bundle of nerve fibers that links the left and right brain hemispheres and that is not fully myelinated or developed in most children until the age of ten (Denckla 1977).

Research shows that hand preference develops as early as the age of three in some children and as late as ten in others. Handedness seems to develop along with the maturation of the nervous system and particularly with the growth of myelin, an insulating matter in the corpus callosum. In immature dyslexic boys, this process is delayed. Myelination of the corpus callosum is also positively correlated with the learning of precise body-movement skills and basic cognitive processes (Herron 1976). Left-handed neuropsychologically immature children have a higher incidence of headaches, dizziness, and sleep problems; they also have greater preschool adjustment and first-grade achievement problems, such as reading disabilities (Trotter 1974). Early studies by Belmont and Birch (1967) show that many young reading-retarded children have a confusion in right-left identification of such things as their own body parts. Also, significant right-left confusion on higher-order perceptual tasks for some children with reading disability was found by Croxen and Lytton (1971). A series of neuropsychological studies by Bakker, Teunissen, and Bosch (1976) conclude that boys are much slower than girls in progressing through these and other successive laterality-reading patterns.

Dyslexic boys take much longer to mature and learn than the girls they must compete with in school. It must be acknowledged that immature children with severe reading disabilities require extra time and special instruction if they are to succeed in school. Since maturational problems in dyslexic children seldom disappear with age or training, good teaching and proper educational organization are continually required if these students are to achieve as much as they can and continue to progress at their own rates.

DEVELOPMENTAL ACHIEVEMENT CLASSES

Schools can be organized so that they improve chances for success and minimize chances for failure. Good organization begins with early identification of learning-handicapped children and realistic provisions for their needs. In most school systems, kindergarten and first-grade children are evaluated for reading readiness. The resulting test information is used for instructional organization and planning.

For example, in one large district, seventy first-grade classes were evaluated with the Lee-Clark Reading Readiness Test in September. Table 10 (Valett 1963, p. 157) shows the expectation of success in reading for these young children; 85 percent have a fair to excellent expectation of success. However, in this district where the average first-grade classroom had thirty-two children, at least five had a poor or very poor expectation of success in reading (Valett 1963).

The Lee-Clark figures, derived from over 2,100 first-grade children in a typical middle class community, are typical of many schools. What should be done with the 15 percent of first-grade children who are already six months or more behind in reading-readiness skills? Of greater concern to parents and teachers of dyslexic children is the question of what would be done to educate the 118 children (mostly boys) who are a year or more behind in basic reading-readiness skills.

A similar twelve-year prospective study of reading retardation in 1,000 children is reported by Bell, Abrahamson, and McRae (1977). They found that poor school achievement can be expected if there is developmental unevenness in auditory, visual-motor, and body skills at the time the child enters school. Differences in children beginning school were substantial: in 508 second-grade children evaluated, reading performance varied from inability to read a single word to a sixth-grade proficiency level. Furthermore, preschool screening instruments were found to be valid and reliable in identifying high-risk children.

As children get older, the spread in reading performance increases. In the typical elementary school, children are grouped by age with little or no consideration given to their performance and achievement in reading. Such grouping puts immature children in competition with those of average and high achievement. A study of over eighteen hundred fourth-grade children (Valett 1963, p. 156) illustrates the increasing spread of achievement in reading vocabulary and reading comprehension. Table 11 shows this spread to be more than six years, ranging from below second-grade to above seventh-grade performance. Even so this table does not reflect the actual extremes

TABLE 10. Lee-Clark Reading Readiness Test

| | Expectation of Success in Reading | | | | |
	Excellent	Good	Fair	Poor	Very Poor
Grade placement	1.5–1.9	1.0–1.4	0.5–0.9	0.0–0.4	0
Delay indicated	None	None	1–5 mo.	6–10 mo.	1 yr. or more
Number of pupils	828	575	468	185	118
Class average	12	8	7	3	2
Percentage distribution	38%	25%	22%	9%	6%

since some children scored on the first-grade level and a few scored on the high tenth-grade level.

Another way to consider the magnitude and importance of individual differences in reading and other academic skills is to contrast the achievement scores of different schools and classes. All educators know that in lower socioeconomic neighborhoods, schools with typical chronological-age class groupings tend to show poor achievement test scores. The scores in Table 12 (Valett 1963, p. 161) are derived from three fourth-grade classes in different schools, *all of which were attempting to follow the same curriculum.*

Fourth-grade children in the low-achieving class were slower learners, much older (due to retentions), and were a year and a half behind in reading comprehension. They were also at least six months behind the fourth-grade curriculum in all other academic subjects.

TABLE 11.   Range of CTMM and CAT* Scores in Fourth-Grade Classes

Grade-Placement Scores	Number of students		Reading Vocabulary	Reading Comprehension
	Language	Nonlanguage		
7.0	IQ: 130 63	IQ: 130 184	95	57
6.7	36	45	56	27
6.3	62	91	75	59
6.0	IQ: 120 61	IQ: 120 81	96	70
5.7	65	67	123	101
5.3	117	99	152	135
5.0	IQ: 110 95	IQ: 110 93	110	132
4.7	111	94	91	127
4.3	171	97	169	164
4.0	IQ: 100 134	IQ: 100 99	117	142
3.7	114	90	212	115
3.3	165	110	209	256
3.0	IQ: 90 117	IQ: 90 77	109	124
2.7	127	68	89	119
2.3	94	92	93	143
2.0	IQ: 80 70	IQ: 80 54	21	42
1.7	207	243	20	23
Total number	1819	1824	1837	1836

*California Test of Mental Maturity and California Achievement Test

But since these are *slow-learning* youngsters, they should not be expected to cope with the regular fourth-grade curriculum. If they are to achieve in reading comprehension, vocabulary, and other skills, they must be provided with opportunities to progress at *their own rates* and must be rewarded (rather than punished) for doing so.

Many schools can be justifiably criticized for producing learning disabilities through poor placement of children and inappropriate instruction. Eysenck (1975) states that failure has been imposed on children by inappropriate methods of teaching that do not take into account innate ability. Studies by Bennett (1976) show that boys with low reading achievement do poorly in regular classes and perform much better in learning situations where they are better motivated and are provided with time to practice appropriate tasks. Extensive work indicates that most students can attain a high level of learning "if instruction is approached sensitively and systematically, if students are helped when and where they have learning difficulty, if they are given sufficient time to achieve mastery, and if there is some clear criterion of what constitutes mastery" (Bloom 1976, p. 4).

It is also necessary for the *entire school* to make provision for mastery and individualized learning. This process should begin with predictive tests in preschool and kindergarten. Special education should be given as soon as it is needed. There are many alternative "developmental achievement" systems that are far more effective in helping young children learn to read than the typical age-grouped class.

In a study of Israeli kibbutz practices, Bettelheim (1969) reports that children are placed in an extended kindergarten from the ages of four to seven. There all of their health, nutritional, and educational

TABLE 12. Range of Achievement Scores in Three Fourth-Grade Classes

Class Ability and Achievement	Age Range	Language I.Q.	Reading Language	Reading Vocabulary	Reading Comprehension	Arithmetic Reasoning	Arithmetic Fundamentals	Mechanical English	Spelling
High	9.0 -9.10	121	111	5.9	6.0	5.5	5.2	4.9	5.9
Average	8.10 -10.8	100	104	4.5	4.0	4.2	4.1	4.3	3.9
Low	8.10 -11.8	76	67	3.4	2.6	3.1	3.3	3.5	3.3

needs are met. In such a setting, low performers are brought up to prevailing peer standards and become highly sociable and competent persons with fewer emotional disturbances than similar children in the United States. Later achievement test results show that these kibbutz children score higher than children in other kinds of schools except for upper-middle-class urban schools with high academic standards. Other studies indicate the value of organizing extended kindergarten or early childhood education programs. These early developmental multiage groups can prevent later learning problems.

Separate classes for young boys and girls have been proposed. Margaret Mead points out that most elementary teachers are women who confront the dilemma of educating boys to be men. In school girls relate easily to women teachers and their values and have another edge over boys in school activities. Furthermore,

> If a boy cries, he is scolded more than a girl who doesn't cry; when she outstrips him, he is told it is even worse than if he had been outstripped by a boy, and yet she may be almost twice his size. . . . side by side they sit in the nursery to be compared on table manners, side by side in school to be compared on neatness and punctuality, as well as reading and writing and arithmetic. She sits and challenges him, and beats him at least half the time and often more than half . . . . as he sits and is beaten he feels it is an intolerable humiliating situation (Mead 1949, p. 314).

Since the preceding words were written, the situation has become even more intolerable for boys. Millions of children are in school who never used to attend at all. Children from various ethnic groups and exceptional children of all kinds who are being "mainstreamed" into "regular programs" are being humiliated. Increasingly, we have great numbers of children who cannot cope with the *traditionally organized* reading program and educational system. For immature, dyslexic children who are forced into this traditional mold, school can become a nightmare of frustration, fear, and failure.

In a review of more than two thousand books and articles on the subject, Maccoby and Jacklin (1974) confirm that boys act out more and have greater visual-spatial and mathematical abilities, whereas girls have greater auditory and verbal abilities. Such differences in school performance might be better provided for by grouping immature boys by themselves. Studies by Lyles (1966) and Kernkamp and Price (1972), among others, demonstrate that boys perform better in reading when grouped separately. A doctoral study by Tregaskis (1972) shows that immature boys with low readiness scores benefit most from all-male groupings and "masculinized reading." Research by Erman (1973) indicates that children prefer teachers of their own sex, and Cascario (1972) reports that young boys taught by males do as well as or better than boys taught by females. These developmental achievement groupings attempt to make the reading process more sensible, meaningful, and relevant to the real needs of immature students. As Smith (1977, p. 395) emphasizes, "Children who can make sense of instruction should learn to read; children confronted by nonsense are bound to fail."

SENSIBLE SCHOOL ORGANIZATION

The only sensible school organization provides for the varied needs of children so that they are taught what they need to know and rewarded for making continuous progress. This goal is best accomplished through the use of special groups and individualized instruction.

Of course, many schools are making serious attempts to adapt to the individual needs of children. One of the most famous models for developmental placement is the Weston and New Haven, Connecticut, Study, which demonstrates the serious overplacement of kindergarten, first, and second-grade children (Ilg and Ames 1965). Readiness tests were used to place these young children in class groups according to their "developmental behavior age" instead of their chronological age. This study recommends that boys' typical six-month lag be considered when placing boys and girls in the same class. Also, children two or more years behind should be in ungraded groups with intensive individualized help. Ilg and Ames believe that accurate behavioral grouping could solve many of the problems that plague teachers and principals alike.

Nongraded grouping by itself may be as ineffective as traditional grouping. For example, the longitudinal study of reading retardation by Bell, Abrahamson, and McRae (1977) suggests that open space, nongraded schools have twice as many reading failures as traditional graded ones (due in part to the distracting influence of open spaces). Also, research by Bennett (1976) indicates that greater progress is made in basic skill achievement through the use of more formal, structured teaching styles and methods. The physical placement of learning-disabled children within schools and class groups requires special structure and organization. Studies by Bakker and Van Rijnsoever (1977) indicate that primary learning-handicapped children achieve best if they are seated in the *middle* of the classroom because of the acoustic-auditory perceptual advantages. Other special arrangements in the physical plant and curricular organization may be required.

The architecture of many new elementary schools reflects concern for the needs of exceptional children. One example is the John O. Tynes Elementary School in Placentia, California, which was built to accommodate nearly eight hundred pupils, many of whom have severe learning problems and handicaps. This school has special libraries, resource and prescriptive therapy rooms, and movable wall partitions that give great flexibility in arranging space. The school is pleasing to the eye, practical, and motivationally exciting.

An example of a special development curriculum is the Fresno Unified School District's POINT program (Montgomery 1971). This Patterned Observation and INTervention program emphasizes teacher observation to determine student strengths and weaknesses and subsequent provision of special instruction. Program officials consulted the Institute of Neurological Sciences of the San Francisco Pacific Medical Center to determine the best design for providing supplemental instruction in critical developmental skills for the younger primary children. Through observation teachers group children according to similar learning styles or strengths. Then they are trained in critical visual, auditory, kinesthetic-motor, visual-motor, and integrative behaviors. Many other school disticts, such as Santa Clara, California, and East Lansing, Michigan, have devised similar programs. These innovative school organization programs attempt to provide for the developmental needs of their students.

Children with severe reading disabilities (or those very young children with high risk of failure in reading) should be grouped according to functional reading achievement. Test scores in reading readiness, vocabulary, phonics, and reading comprehension, as well as teacher observation should all be considered in grouping classes. Of course, grouping for reading instruction should occur only for an hour or so a day; children can then be regrouped for instruction in arithmetic and for general social interaction. As we have seen, in most cases boys should be in reading classes on lower levels than girls of the same age. In some schools, it may be best to separate boys from girls at the earlier developmental levels of instruction. Where achievement grouping in reading is used, it is suggested that the kindergarten-primary years be divided into fifteen reading instruction achievement groups, while the upper grades be organized into twelve achievement levels as Table 13 shows.

Such a flexible achievement grouping for basic instruction in reading would need modification to meet the varying needs of students. The number of students on each level might vary considerably, as would instructional materials, books, and other resources. The important thing is that sensible provision be made for all children to learn to read at their own rates, without fear of failure or undue frustration. This would eventually reduce the number of reading-disabled children and would certainly minimize the organizational factors that exacerbate dyslexic tendencies. But even with achievement reading groups for all children, educators must still provide supplemental prescriptive instruction for dyslexic children.

SUPPLEMENTAL PRESCRIPTIVE INSTRUCTION

When children begin to fail in reading, they immediately should get additional help and special instruction. The first step is to make sure the child has been properly placed in the most appropriate reading achievement group. Since children are frequently overplaced in all kinds of groups and classes, it may be that a child with difficulties should move to a group in accord with his or her developmental reading skills. If failure continues, such children should then be placed in special remedial reading center groups for two or more hours a day until the essential skills are mastered. For example, in the public schools of Horsholm, Denmark, such children are placed in small clinical groups of three or four. During a twelve-week period they meet all morning in a separate room to review and develop critical reading skills. This approach is highly successful and most children are able to acquire missing skills and then return to regular reading classes and subgroups.

TABLE 13. **Reading Achievement Level Placement**

Pre-School Developmental Levels	Kindergarten Readiness Levels	Primary (Grades 1-3) Reading Levels	Upper Elementary (Grades 4-7) Reading Levels
1, 2, 3	4, 5, 6	7–15	16–27

Sometimes it is wise to retain the child in a particular reading group, level, or program. If a child has been sick or absent a great deal, he or she cannot have been adequately exposed to learning opportunities. Careful evaluation, using instruments such as Light's Retention Scale (Light 1977) along with observation and criterion task analysis, is necessary to determine if and when retention is wise. If the child has been diagnosed as dyslexic, retention by itself seldom provides the required special education. This can be done only by supplemental special educators working in special rooms and clinics.

Special educators should conduct intensive individual and small-group instruction for dyslexic children in school clinics, regular classrooms, and homes. They should provide remedial training in critical attentional, perceptual, cognitive, verbal, semantic, and syntactic skills recommended by Jensen (1969), Vellutino (1977), and others. Special educators must help administrators and regular teachers in the proper group placement (or mainstreaming) of dyslexic children. Also, they should help schools design alternative organizational strategies to improve learning. In addition, these diagnostic-prescriptive specialists must teach dyslexic children to compensate by using their strengths and talents to their advantage. Bogan (1975) suggests that special programs should provide those with right-hemispheric dominance increased opportunities to excel in the arts, mechanics, and other areas requiring their visual-spatial skills and abilities.

Specialists working with dyslexic children must work closely with parents. Parents need practical suggestions and materials for helping their children at home. We have already discussed several successful programs of parental involvement. In some cases, it is wise to engage parents in systematic home instruction of their children. For example, the Trenton, New Jersey, schools have developed the New Approach Method to reading—a tape-recorded series that parents use at home with young children. With reinforcement from parents and support from professionals, children as young as four can be successfully taught readiness and beginning primary reading skills. Many other similar individual approaches may be used to help dyslexics acquire the skills and confidence they need to learn.

Every public school should have a special developmental-remedial reading clinic staffed by a reading specialist. In addition, every average-sized school should have at least one special educator who provides supplemental intensive prescriptive teaching for children with learning disabilities. The special educator should work out of a learning resource center equipped with many of the instructional programs and aids mentioned in this book. Both of these educational specialists should have an adequate budget to obtain new and necessary learning materials, including sensory, perceptual, language, and cognitive development materials. These specialists should elicit the involvement of parents, peer tutors, community volunteers, and other teachers in the program. It is essential that once a prescriptive reading program has been designed for a child, all persons involved be informed and consistently reinforce desirable reading behaviors whenever and wherever they occur. Many illustrations of successful behavior modification strategies to reinforce reading skills are given by Axelrod (1977) and others.

Schools and special education programs must become more accountable to parents and the general public. With the passage of Public Law 94-142, all handicapped children *must* be provided full opportunities for education everywhere in this country. Most states have devised legislation to carry out and supplement federal law. This legislation has resulted in master plans for special education that address needs of dyslexic and other learning-disabled children. All of these laws demand that school administrators and special teachers devise systematic screening, referral, and evaluation systems. The first step in screening and evaluation is to observe the child carefully and record specific learning problems. One example of a record form designed to meet this purpose is given on the next page. Federal law also requires that an Individual Educational Plan (IEP) be written for each dyslexic child identified and receiving special funding. These plans must be periodically evaluated for effectiveness and possible revisions.

The new California Master Plan for Special Education and Assembly Bill 1250 requires school superintendents to submit annual evaluations of all special education programs. Special individualized education is provided for all persons from the ages of three through twenty-two. The California Education Code specifies that educationally handicapped pupils are eligible for admission to special education programs if, among other things,

> The learning or behavioral disorders are specific learning disabilities in the psychological, mental, or physiological processes involved in understanding or in using spoken or written language. Such learning disabilities include, but are not limited to, those sometimes referred to as perceptual handicaps, minimal brain dysfunction, dyslexia, dyscalculia, dysgraphia, or communication disorders (Title V, Chapter 2, Article 3).

In California, Title V states that an educational assessment service team shall determine the content of each individualized education pro-

BEHAVIOR OBSERVATION RECORD

(To meet requirements of California Administrative Code, Title V, Article 3, Section 3231)

Student observed _____ Birthdate _____ School _____

This observation was requested by _____ on the date of _____

1. Teacher Description of student's school difficulty which is to be observed:

2. Observed Behaviors:

Date	Place	Time	Instructional objective(s)	Learning materials and tasks involved	Behavioral actions observed (baseline behaviors)

3. Factors to Be Considered (What observed "environmental factors and peer and teacher interactions" may possibly be contributing to this student's school difficulty?)

4. Assistance:

a. What "specific steps have been taken to assist this student in the area of his or her school difficulty?"

b. What was the observed effectiveness and/or results of this assistance?

5. Recommended Follow-up:

a. Priority educational goals or instructional objectives:

b. Instructional materials, programs, placement, etc.:

c. Positive reinforcement to be used:

d. Other comments and recommendations:

Observer's signature   Date gram and make appropriate placement recommendations. For dyslexic and other learning-handicapped students, this initial plan must include all of the following:

1. clearly defined instructional goals to (a) reduce the handicapping effect of the child's disability, (b) specify the remedial instruction required, (c) enhance strengths

2. recommendations for educational approaches, methods, services, or specific interventions that can be carried out within the regular or special program recommended

3. recommendations, when indicated, for a specific differential program or grouping, or modification of an existing class or group, to accommodate a particular student or to meet his or her educational needs

4. recommendations regarding necessary ancillary services to be provided by the school, parent or guardian, or community, wherever such recommendations are essential for the proper maintenance of a program appropriate to the needs of the student.

This plan must be reduced to specific educational objectives by the teacher responsible for the special education program in which the dyslexic child is placed. Objectives must include expected learning behavior skills, anticipated levels of attainment, and criterion methods, measures, or tests to determine whether or not the objectives have been realized. One example of an Individual Educational Plan form appears on page 262.

There are many different ways supplemental prescriptive instruction can be provided in the schools. Three commonly used models are outlined in Table 14. In Model A the teacher has planned half-days for teaching cognitive, psychomotor, and affective lessons. In Model B the teacher follows the same organizational plan every day with regular classroom visits and supplemental tutoring. Model C is a combination of the other two plans and provides four weekly periods for peer tutoring. The important common characteristic in these plans is the provision for meeting the learning objectives of dyslexic or learning-handicapped children in *both* the regular and special education setting.

SUMMARY

Dyslexic children need schools organized to permit and encourage them to learn and progress at their own rates. Traditional grouping based on age is detrimental to dyslexic and other exceptional children.

INDIVIDUAL EDUCATIONAL PLAN FOR DYSLEXIC STUDENTS

Student's Name		Birthdate		Sex

School	Special Education Program

Regular Teacher	Special Teacher

Instructional objectives	Priority	Anticipated levels of attainment (minimal performance expectations)	Instructional strategies (placement, materials)	Criterion measures (tests, instruments)
Sensory/psychomotor skills:				
Auditory/visual-perceptual skills:				
Language skills:				
Reading skills:				
Conceptual/thinking skills:				
Social/affective skills:				
Other:				

Signature(s):		Date	Date of anticipated evaluation and revision

The evidence is overwhelming that significant maturational differences exist among children. These differences have great educational implications that can be ignored no longer by responsible school officials and an increasingly concerned public. Boys mature more slowly than girls in many respects, as is shown by their significantly slower acquisition of verbal, language, and reading-readiness skills. Young boys must be grouped so that they can develop these critical skills without unfair competition, humiliation, frustration, and relative failure.

All children should be placed in classes and learning groups according to their functional achievement. Developmental achievement grouping in reading is essential for dyslexic children and should be required in all public schools. Whenever possible, male teachers should be assigned to work with classes or groups of dyslexic boys.

TABLE 14. Models for Organizing Learning-Handicapped Programs

	A					B					C				
	M	Tu	W	Th	F	M	Tu	W	Th	F	M	Tu	W	Th	F
A.M.	Cognitive lessons	Cognitive lessons	Psychomotor lessons	Regular classroom visits/tutoring	Group/individual affective lessons	Individual cognitive lessons ... Individual and group psychomotor lessons					Psychomotor lessons ... Cognitive lessons ... Group affective lesson				Regular classroom visits and tutoring
P.M.	Individual affective lessons	Regular classroom visits/tutoring	Cognitive lessons	Cognitive lessons	Psychomotor lessons	Regular classroom visits and supplemental tutoring ... Affective lesson discussion group					Group cognitive lessons ... Peer tutoring				

Whatever the school organization, dyslexic children will require supplemental prescriptive education by qualified special teachers who provide intensive developmental-remedial instruction in resource centers and clinics. These specialists must work closely with regular teachers and involve parents.

Every dyslexic child should have an Individual Educational Plan devised to meet his or her needs. This plan should include instructional objectives and learning strategies. All teachers concerned need to be aware of this plan, as must students and parents. These individual learning objectives need to be reevaluated periodically and revised accordingly. Schools should be held accountable for providing appropriate education for dyslexic children.

DISCUSSION QUESTIONS AND ACTIVITIES

1. Define *education*. Formulate your own educational goals for dyslexic children.

2. List some stress differences between males and females that make boys more physically and psychologically vulnerable.

3. Why have IQ-test norms been manipulated to make scores of males more equal to those of females?

4. Outline several language advantages of young girls that lead to superior reading scores.

5. What evidence do we have that dyslexic boys are delayed in neuropsychological maturation?

6. Discuss the extent to which dyslexic children might be expected to catch up with their nondyslexic peers.

7. What should be done with children designated as "very poor achieving" by kindergarten and first-grade reading-readiness tests?

8. Survey the spread of reading achievement scores on standardized tests used in your school. What proportion of primary students scoring in the lowest 15 percent are boys?

9. What are the different kinds of reading groups and school placement patterns that are used in your district? How are severely reading-disabled children grouped?

10. List and discuss three different reading-readiness and achievement tests that are used (or could be used) in your school.

11. To what extent might female teachers be inappropriate instructors of dyslexic boys?

12. Describe a sensible school organization plan for dyslexic children.

13. Demonstrate and discuss one developmental-readiness program or model that might help prevent learning disabilities.

14. Assume you are a diagnostic-prescriptive special educator working with dyslexic children in a public elementary school. Design and outline an ideal program. Show how, when, and where you would use your time.

15. Discuss local policies and procedures pertaining to exceptional children and the writing of Individual Educational Plans.

16. Make up an Individual Education Plan form as shown in this chapter. Use a student you know as a subject.

17. What could your school district do to improve services and programs for dyslexic children?

Progress, therefore, is not an accident, but a necessity.

Herbert Spencer

CHAPTER FOURTEEN

Prognosis and Expectations

There is considerable evidence that dyslexia is a neuropsychological processing disorder and that much can be done to help dyslexic children learn to read. Because harassed teachers and anxious parents need support and encouragement, we have tried here to take a positive approach with few qualifications.

However, it needs to be strongly stated that most research in this field is incomplete. The neurological, psychological, linguistic, and related sciences are still too immature to provide firm direction for educational practice. Although research and interest in dyslexia has increased dramatically over the last few years, results are still tentative or inconclusive. Therefore, special education and other treatment for dyslexic children must be perceived as applied clinical attempts of an ongoing experimental nature. As such, treatment for dyslexics will continue to change with time and experience. As in all fields, progress in research and work with dyslexic children is not an accident but a necessity. And, as Herbert Spencer implied, progress itself is dependent on continued effort, research, and development.

The now vast literature on dyslexia is replete with programs, experiments, and studies that have failed or have been found invalid. We have dealt sparingly with such material, but the reader who is about to design or implement any applied educational program will want to go directly to the sources listed in the bibliography here and to such supplementary material as may be of special interest.

In this final chapter, we will consider the prognosis and expectations for the treatment and education of dyslexic children. Real progress in research and education has been made and will continue. We will first consider this progress by contrasting some case studies and methods of the 1920s with a contemporary study. The older work is drawn from the classical reports of Samuel Orton. The contemporary case summary on a boy named James illustrates a number of current approaches and techniques.

CLASSICAL ILLUSTRATIONS

In 1925 Dr. Samuel Orton published an article, "Word-Blindness in School Children," that has become a classic in the literature on dyslexia and specific language disabilities. In this article, Orton reviews a study of several children whose chief difficulty was in learning to read. Two of these children he diagnosed as having "congenital word-blindness," which today we refer to as developmental dyslexia.

One child, Clark C., ten years old, had a Stanford-Binet IQ score of 102 but presented some highly unusual characteristics. He was repeating the third grade and was described by his teachers as "very dull" with poor reading ability and retarded motor reactions. When reading directly from a textbook he made constant reversal and omission errors, even in such words as *nod, bend,* and *dance.* But when he viewed the same text in a mirror he could read a sentence of fifteen words promptly and correctly. This is Clark's description of himself: "Mother says there is something funny about me because you could read anything to me and I'd get it right away, but if I read it myself I couldn't get it" (Orton 1937/1966, p. 29).

From cases such as this, Orton became convinced that many "word-blind" children were of essentially normal intelligence but suffered from congenital developmental neurological immaturity in brain lateralization that resulted in reversals and mirror reading.

Orton's most striking case was a boy sixteen years and two months old, whom he referred to as M.P. On the Stanford-Binet intelligence test this boy had an IQ score of 71, which Orton considered to be invalid due to the boy's special disability. M.P. had good visual memory and was able to discuss the adjustments of bearings in an automobile engine with great accuracy. On a retest of the Binet his score was 86, while on several mechanical tests he scored on the superior level. However his reading, writing, and spelling were all immature and labored. M.P. had an extremely short memory span for a series of letter sounds. Although he could read words more easily when they were broken down into syllables, his retention was quite limited. His faulty association of sounds with letters led to many substitutions and distortions. M.P. tended to reverse parts or all of a word: he perceived the word *gray* as *gary*.

Orton instituted special training in sound-symbol association, synthesis, and sequencing. He made use of M.P.'s strong visual sense and his ability to translate ideas into speech. A combined speaking, reading, and writing program was developed and used. Finally M.P. learned to read and write a few words correctly, but fluency in association never developed, and both oral and silent reading remained very difficult for him. Phonic training resulted in some improvement, but the long-run prognosis was poor.

We do not know what happened to M.P. but he probably dropped out of school, went to work, and merged with the great number of other slow-learning and reading-disabled persons in the community.

In the 1920s it was unusual to provide children like M.P. with any form of special education. M.P. was fortunate to have received any remedial instruction since auditory decoding and phonics training were not widespread in the public schools. Gradually phonics instruction has become the rule, and almost all children have been exposed to formal phonics in the primary grades. Special education of all kinds has become widespread, and the most common remedial procedures have followed the phonics model initiated by Orton. At the present time other forms of special education seem more promising.

CONTEMPORARY APPROACHES

James is a good-looking fifteen-year-old with a long history of reading and language problems. When he began kindergarten he had very limited language skills and was referred for special education. Psycholinguistic evaluation disclosed extremely poor auditory discrimination and atypical motor phonetic ability. On the nonverbal Leiter International Performance Scale, James scored in a borderline retarded range with an IQ score of 67. With a diagnosis of developmental aphasia, James was placed in a special class for children with severe language disabilities.

Initial psychometric scores disclosed that James was a visual learner. He had always done well on both the WISC and the ITPA visual closure, completion, and organization tasks; his most recent WISC Picture Completion subtest score was 14, significantly above average. James adapted well to special education and gradually learned to read through a combination of experiential sensory-motor activities and compensatory visual word cues.

James is a well-liked and friendly boy, and he has slowly acquired a fairly good self-concept. His general view of the school and his world is positive and outgoing. In the middle elementary grades his expressive language had developed to the point where he was transferred to a nongraded learning-handicapped class, which he has attended for the last several years.

Recently increasing emphasis has been placed on development of James's auditory abilities through concentrated lessons using the Auditory Discrimination in Depth (ADD), SRA Corrective Reading, and DISTAR Programs. James has also been involved in some sensory-motor integration programs and activities. His progress has been slow and labored as illustrated by continued reversals in the ADD lessons and many substitution errors in the SRA Corrective Reading Program. Although still below his measured potential James has made progress and is now reading on a functional fourth-grade level.

Some of James's most recent test scores are summarized on the psychoeducational profile on the next page. His WISC Performance Scale subtests have a mean score of 9.6 (average), but borderline performance discrepancies are found in both the Block Design (visual-motor synthesis) and Coding (speed and accuracy) subtests. All of his WISC Verbal Scale subtest scores are below average with an achievement expectancy of low fifth grade.

Interestingly, his ITPA auditory deficiencies remain significant problems, although he has demonstrated improvement in these areas. He has always been extremely poor in auditory closure (putting syllables, blends, and words together), and although he has acquired some of these skills through special training and experience, this area is still of critical concern. Although it is not reflected on the profile, part of James's auditory difficulty is due to mixed laterality and hemispheric confusion. James appears to be consistently right-sided, but on a dichotic listening test he demonstrated a left-ear advantage (LEA) of

PSYCHOEDUCATIONAL PROFILES

Name	James		Grade	LHB		CA	15 yrs. 2 mos.	

			Profile of standard scores				
	Skills and abilities	Very low	Below average	Average	Above average	Very high
WISC Performance Scores:						
PS IQ: 104	Picture completion				14	
MA: 15 yrs. 5 mos.	Picture arrangement			9		
	Block design		7			
Grade expect: 10.2	Object assembly			11		
	Coding		7			
WISC Verbal Scores:						
V IQ: 72	Information		6			
MA: 10 yrs. 8 mos.	Similarities		5			
	Arithmetic	4				
Grade expect: 5.3	Vocabulary	4				
	Comprehension		6			
	Digit span		6			
ITPA Scores:	Visual closure			36		
	Auditory closure	8 ⟶ 27				
	Auditory reception	16→24				
	Auditory association	16→24				
WRAT Reading:	Sight vocabulary Grade P.: 2.9	−1%				
Spache Reading:	Sight vocabulary Grade P.: 3.9	X				
	Oral paragraphs Grade P.: Low Fourth		X			
	Oral comprehension Grade P.: High Fifth			X		

Discrepancy between reading achievement and potential: $1\frac{1}{2}$ to 6 years.

Strengths: Visual organization and comprehension.

Weaknesses: Auditory sequencing and closure. Reversals, mixed laterality—right-handed with left-ear advantage.

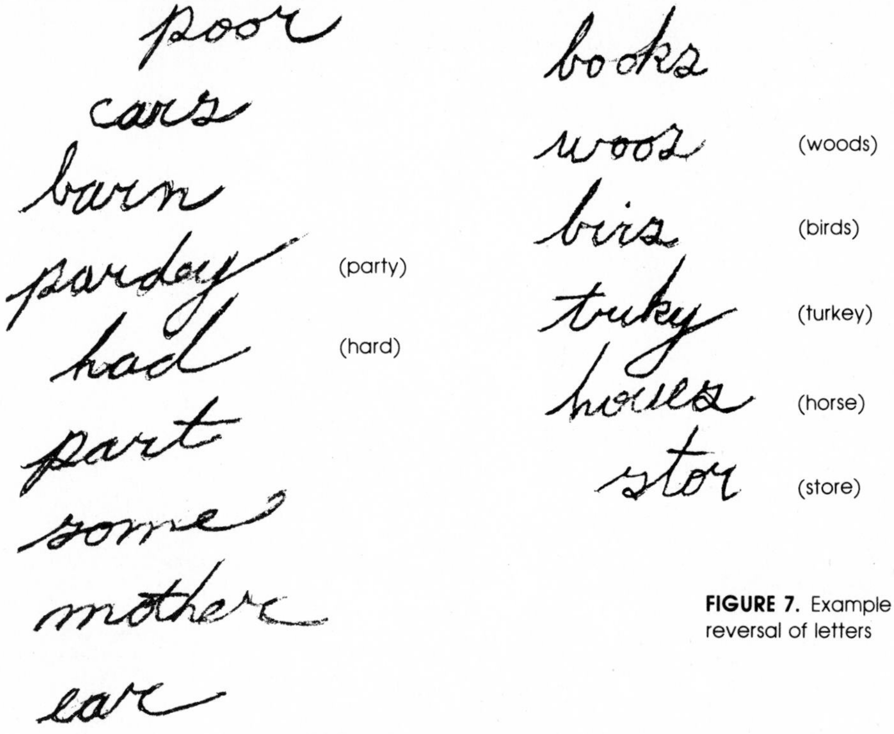

poor

cars

barn

pardey (party)

had (hard)

part

some

mother

ear

books

woos (woods)

birs (birds)

truky (turkey)

hoires (horse)

stor (store)

FIGURE 7. Example of omission and reversal of letters

eighteen points over his right ear — evidence that he processes language more efficiently in his right hemisphere.

The Dichotic Listening Survey on page 18 was used with James. He first listened to music in his left ear and heard digit-sound-word sequences simultaneously in his right ear. Then the procedure was reversed. James did fairly well on digit sequences and was able to repeat six digits heard in his right ear and five digits in the left ear. However, in repeating letter-sound sequences he made many more errors using his right ear. He repeated the sequence *v-e-l-r-c* as *d-e-r-l-c*. Many of his oral and written errors were reversals, distortions, and omissions, although he was able to sequence letter-sounds much better when listening to them through his left ear. With the left ear he repeated *sh-ly-er-ic* correctly, but *en-sh-ly-er* heard in his right ear was rendered as *en-sl-* (omissions). These and other tests reflect James's left-hemispheric language-processing disability. James's relatively superior visual and visual-motor skills are reflected in his writing and drawing. His handwriting is fairly clear, as can be seen in the organization and style of the spelling words above. But again, his difficulty with auditory memory and synthesis appears in the omission and reversal of letters. See Figure 7.

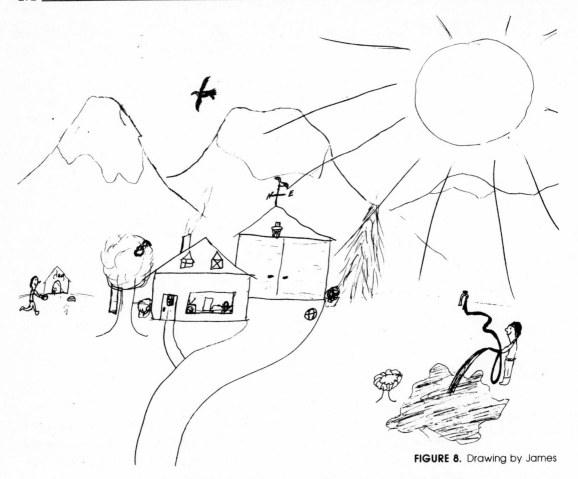

FIGURE 8. Drawing by James

James's poor auditory memory and sequencing difficulties surface in other kinds of writing tasks. Part of the dichotic listening test involves listening to digit and letter sequences and then writing them in reverse order. Although James was able to write clearly, he often failed to give the correct sequence. When he heard two-element sequences such as *2-5* and *b-k,* he was able to reverse them correctly and write *5-2* and *k-b,* but as soon as three or more digits or letters occurred, James made reversals, omissions, and substitutions that support the other evidence of left-hemisphere auditory processing immaturity.

James's strength in visual organization and comprehension is also reflected in his drawing and coloring. He enjoys drawing pictures.

Figure 8 is a typical drawing by James. Many of his pictures contain a shining sun, good perspective, proper proportion, and interesting detail. His drawing is further evidence of a right-hemisphere visual-

TRENDS AND
TRANSITIONS

spatial skill superiority and thus substantiates the highly significant differences between his verbal and performance scale IQ scores on the WISC.

As we have seen, James is a developmental dyslexic with left-hemispheric immaturity including specific auditory synthesis dysfunctions. After years of special education he is well adapted socially and has learned to read. Continued special education and development will be required throughout his high school training. If he is fortunate, he will receive some on-the-job training designed to make use of his good visual-spatial abilities.

There is a great difference between the special education given M.P. over fifty years ago and that provided for James. James had the advantage of receiving several kinds of special education beginning in the primary grades. Differences also exist in the quality of diagnostic-prescriptive tests, instructional materials, and related services that were and are now available for dyslexic children. Of course many things are still lacking, and although the prognosis for James is fairly good at this time, much remains to be done for him in high school.

TRENDS AND TRANSITIONS

Research, technology, and new educational methods all indicate that we are in a transitional state in the diagnosis and treatment of dyslexic and other learning-disabled children. There is a widening awareness of this class of disability and an increasing provision of special educational services for these children in public schools.

Most of these services are dependent upon some form of systematic screening, identification, and evaluation of dyslexic children. The trend is toward earlier screening and intervention beginning on the preschool level. There is also a growing movement to provide special education throughout all the school years and into adulthood.

Danenhower (1972) reports on one successful program for teaching adults with language disabilities. In this program a group of unemployed adults were carefully evaluated; more than 26 percent presented evidence of developmental dyslexia. Some new screening instruments were devised in this project and proved to be very effective. This remedial model is a good illustration of emerging adult special education programs.

Diagnostic and evaluation procedures are being refined so that they relate more directly to prescriptive interventions. Although we still do not have a test procedure that identifies dyslexia with certainty, evidence is accumulating that will eventually be integrated into more meaningful diagnostic-prescriptive reports. For example, Wolf's (1967) experimental investigation of dyslexic boys shows that their most significant error on standardized reading tests was substitutions. On the WISC they had low Maze and Digit Span scores and higher than normal Picture Completion scores. Another highly discriminating measure (.0001) was their poor rhythm as evidenced on the Seashore Rhythm Test. Other investigators report similar findings.

Recent trends are toward new approaches to diagnosis. For example, much research has established that learning-disabled poor readers have significant trouble in focusing on a learning task, sustaining attention, and maintaining field independence from distracting environmental stimuli. These findings have been confirmed through experiments on selective attention, such as that by Hallahan, Gajar, Cohen, and Tarver (1978). Now the trend is to research instructional and treatment methodologies, such as verbal rehearsal strategies, modeling, and other ways of teaching children to think (Valett 1978). Related research on dichotic listening, biofeedback, behavioral/task analysis has resulted in several new and innovative diagnostic-prescriptive approaches.

We have also made progress in understanding the importance of lateral dominance in learning to read. This has been the single most controversial subject in the history of dyslexia, and we can expect the arguments to continue with new research findings on right- and left-brain functions and new educational programs designed to develop or "educate" the whole brain. Bakker (1973) aptly summarizes a number of current studies. He concludes that young children whose sight word perception (and visual/spatial organization) is prominent read well without marked dominance, but with increasing age, and as greater fluency and comprehension are demanded, good reading is associated with increasing dominance. As we have seen, left-hemispheric dominance in most persons results in improved language performance, although Bakker concludes that it is not important which hemisphere eventually dominates.

There is also a trend toward the use of increasing instrumentation in both diagnosis and special education. The experiments of Tomatis (1972) with audio-vocal feedback and filtered sounds resulted in the creation of a device called the "electronic ear." Special earphones increased sounds to the right ear, and children then spoke better and more eagerly and improved their behavior and reading as well. This work shows that developing right-ear preference improves left-hemispheric lateralization and dominance. Undoubtedly instruments of this kind will be refined further and used in both diagnostic work and prescriptive education.

Similar advances have been made in the use of biofeedback. Satterfield and Dawson (1971) found that hyperkinetic children had lower basal skin conductiveness with smaller galvanic skin responses (GSRs) than ordinary children. In the last few years many special psychoeducational treatment programs have been devised by Valett (1974) and others to help such children learn muscular inhibition, relaxation, and self-control. One example of innovative treatment is the use of alpha training with a dyslexic adolescent. O'Malley and Comers (1972) found that such a program significantly increased (.0001) visually evoked response amplitudes in the left hemisphere and improved performance. In a related study on dichotic auditory vigilance during feedback-enhanced EEG alpha training, Kaszniak (1973) discovered decreased peripheral perceptual awareness during alpha with a corresponding improvement in attention and better results on dichotic listening tasks. In the years to come, we can expect greater use of biofeedback in psychoeducational treatment.

There is also a movement toward "whole brain" education that stresses the integration of left-right brain operations. Duane and Rawson (1974) review the research on reading, perception, and language and conclude that children who are not too handicapped linguistically and who are taught with well-planned phonics programs tend to make good progress from the start. But the dyslexic child with psycholinguistic processing and integrational deficiencies must receive special forms of stimulation and education in order to learn and develop. Gillingham (1968) was among the first to propose special training in which all possible linkages between visual, auditory, and kinesthetic sensory impressions (or "engrams") are formed and integrated. Since then many others have contributed to the advancement of multisensory special education. Karnes (1964) has compiled data on dyslexia programs that emphasize simultaneous use of different sensory modalities.

Another emerging trend is toward the increased use of mental imagery and conscious cognitive operations in the treatment of dyslexic children. For example, Oliver (1969) suggests that children be taught to close their eyes and imagine scenes from a paragraph or story they have selected, or that they describe, enact, or draw a scene from the story after it is read aloud by the teacher. Through this process, children achieve fuller integration and meaningful closure. Robbins and Sibley (1976) advocate the use of art activities for exceptional children and suggest art is "symbolic speech" that can be used to stimulate total communication. Visual imagery, symbolic thinking, and spatial organization are important brain functions that contribute to the reading process. The continued development of holistic educational programs stressing right- and left-brain integration should result in new approaches to remedial education.

EDUCATIONAL IMPLICATIONS

Although it is still much too early to propose "principles" of neuropsychological education, some functional guidelines have emerged after fifty years of research and practice.

These guidelines for the special education of dyslexic children are summarized below.

1. Observe. Carefully observe the student's functional reading performance. Establish his or her baseline reading performance relative to criterion reading tasks and tests.

2. Evaluate. Systematically assess, evaluate, and diagnose both reading and neuropsychological dysfunctions.

3. Target objectives. Specify the priority behavior objectives in the psychomotor, cognitive, and affective domains. Indicate why you believe fulfilling the objectives will help the child to learn to read.

4. Relax. Begin teaching the child to relax using progressive relaxation techniques, creative imagination, and autosuggestion.

5. Teach multisensory lessons. Carefully plan, design, and use multisensory methods for integrating auditory (listening to sound patterns), oral (verbalizing, repeating sounds, and identifying concepts), visual (visual feedback and confirmation of integrated auditory-oral sequences), and kinesthetic (reinforcement by tracing or writing language symbols) modalities. Provide special prescriptive education as follows:

   • sensory-integration and vestibular training
   • focused attention and figure-ground differentiation
   • visual tracking and coordination
   • temporal order rhythmic training of letter/sound symbols
   • right ear amplification and feedback exercises
   • syllabication with kinesthetic reinforcement

- formal phonics and auditory training
- neuropsychological impress fluency training
- creative mental imagery and cognitive strategies

6. Motivate. Develop motivation through self-monitoring and reinforcement, positive assertion, improved diet, and systematic social rewards and privileges. Establish cooperative home/school programs.

7. Evaluate and redesign. Periodically consult concerned persons, then examine and redesign your educational strategies.

SUMMARY

In the future we should expect progress in the diagnosis and education of dyslexic children. Such progress, though, is not automatic but depends upon the concerted and cooperative endeavors of professionals of all kinds and parents.

We can anticipate that ongoing research will result in many new psychoeducational applications. With the rapid developments in computer-assisted instruction, nutritional and biochemical intervention and management, biofeedback, auditory training programs and devices, attention training, the use of visual imagery, and cognitive strategies (to mention just a few), dyslexic persons of all ages will learn and function more effectively.

We need the determination to *use* the results of emerging research and technology. But most public schools are slow to change, lack innovation, and lag considerably behind private endeavors. Parents, school board members, and educators must increase their cooperative efforts to design and institute new systems of education in which all children can make continuous progress at their own rates of learning, and in which dyslexic and other learning-disabled children receive appropriate diagnostic-prescriptive education as soon and as long as is needed.

A healthy skepticism concerning both old and new approaches to dyslexic children should continue among persons working in this field. This attitude is most constructively displayed in well-designed programs requiring accountability and evaluation. If we maintain such a pragmatic approach and positive attitude, the prognosis for dyslexic children is certainly fair, perhaps even good.

DISCUSSION QUESTIONS AND ACTIVITIES

1. Select a research study that you feel is questionable. Read the original study and discuss it orally.

2. Discuss Clark C.'s strange ability to mirror-read whole sentences correctly.

3. Discuss the similarities and differences between M.P. and James.

4. Examine the ITPA auditory subtest items and design some instructional tasks and lessons for children, such as James, who have significantly low scores.

5. Have someone administer the Dichotic Listening Survey (page 18) to you and determine your ear preference.

6. Design a remedial spelling lesson for James using the words listed on page 271. Explain how and why you would proceed to teach him these specific words.

7. Visit a local school and write a constructive report describing their program for educating dyslexic children.

8. Outline the major diagnostic characteristics of dyslexic children.

9. To what extent is lateral dominance an important factor in learning to read?

10. What is alpha training?

11. Design a mental imagery lesson for helping a child learn to read. Use the lesson, discuss your results, and suggest how the lesson could have been improved.

12. Select a recent research article on the education of dyslexic children and write a critique.

13. What might you do to help improve the education of dyslexic children in your school or community?

Appendixes

Glossary

acetylcholine (Ach)   a chemical vital to proper neural functioning and synaptic transmission.

agnosia   inability to recognize the form and nature of persons and things through usual auditory or tactile stimulation.

agraphia   loss of writing ability.

alexia   loss of acquired reading ability due to brain impairment.

amblyopia (lazy eye)   condition in which form perception is disturbed within the cortex due to unequal refractive error in crossed eyes.

amphetamine   a central nervous system stimulant frequently used with hyperactive children in the form of dextroamphetamine.

angular gyrus   a folded convolution in part of the lower parietal lobe where memory patterns of written symbols are stored.

anterior   referring to the front part or zone as opposed to the posterior.

aphasia   loss of acquired speech and language.

apraxia   the loss of the ability to perform skilled acts due to brain injury.

articulation   the pronunciation of words.

ataxia   loss of muscle coordination.

auditory   pertaining to hearing.

axon   the part of the neuron that transmits impulses from the cell.

cerebellum   a part of the lower hindbrain concerned with coordination of voluntary movement, posture, and equilibrium.

cerebral dominance   primary control by one side of the brain.

cerebral palsy   involuntary motions due to injury to the motor areas of the brain.

cerebrum   the upper-front part of the brain, which is concerned with conscious processes.

choreiform movements   irregular, spasmodic movements of parts of the body.

cognition   referring to mental processes of knowing or becoming knowledgeable.

congenital   a condition that exists from conception or birth.

consonant   a sound produced by stopping or slowing the passage of air: for example, *b, d, f, s.*

contingencies   the possible consequences of behaving in a certain way.

corpus callosum   the midbrain nerve tissue that joins the left and right hemispheres.

cortex   the top layer of the brain covering the hemispheres.

decoding   the process of interpreting sounds and symbols.

dendrite   the part of the neuron that picks up the stimulus and transmits it to the cell.

desensitization   overcoming excessive sensitivity to anxiety-producing situations through gradual exposure, assurance, and reeducation.

developmental dysphasia excessive maturational delay in the acquisition of speech and expressive language.

developmental immaturity significantly slow rate of growth and total human development

diagnostic-prescriptive education learning tasks and activities derived from systematic individual observation and evaluation.

dichotic listening a testing technique in which earphones deliver different sounds to each ear.

digraph a pair of letters representing a single sound.

dysacusis a hearing dysfunction in which all noises produce sensations of discomfort.

dysarthria extreme difficulty in articulation.

dysgraphia developmental disability in writing.

dyslexia significant developmental delay in reading due to neuropsychological processing deficiencies.

dysphasia significant difficulty in speaking due to brain damage.

echolalia the mechanical imitation and repetition of speech.

electroencephalograph (EEG) an apparatus that records the electrical activity of the brain: useful in diagnosing lesions and tumors.

encoding the understanding and correct usage of language forms and expressions.

feedback the process giving back immediate information on behavioral responses in order that the person may develop greater awareness for modifying his or her future behavior.

focused arousal ability of the brain to focus and concentrate on relevant stimuli.

frontal lobe the front part of the cerebral cortex containing major association areas for thinking and planning.

functional reading the ability to read commonly encountered printed material (signs, newspapers, menus).

gestalt (German, "form") used here to mean viewing a pattern or event as a whole.

glia the supporting fibrous network of cells in the brain and spinal cord.

grammar the standard usage, organization, and rules of language.

grapheme a written or printed sound symbol or letter form.

graphesthenia identification of letters and words "written" on the skin.

haptic referring to the sense of touch.

Hawthorne effect referring to a famous experiment that showed mere change in a person's regular work routine can produce results originally attributed to more special treatment interventions.

hemiplegia paralysis of one side of the body because of brain damage to the opposite hemisphere.

hertz (Hz) unit of measurement of wave frequency (meaning cycles-per-second).

hippocampus a nerve tract in the forebrain that figures in the sense of smell and in the regulation of the internal body organs.

hypoglycemia an abnormally low concentration of sugar in the blood resulting in fatigue and inattention.

idiom as used here, the language of a particular group.

intelligence the general ability to solve problems of living.

language a symbolic code for communication of ideas, feelings, and experiences.

laterality either right- or left-hemispheric dominance of the cerebral cortex.

learning disability a highly significant discrepancy between a person's specific functional ability and measured potential for acquiring and using information and skills essential to problem solving.

lesion a wound, injury, or pathological change in body tissue.

limbic system the central areas of the brain involved in the regulation of emotional and motivational behavior.

maturation the process of natural growth and development.

mediational processes the associative and integrative mental operations occuring between the reception and the expression of sensation, though, and language.

medulla oblongata the prolongation of the spinal cord into the brain.

mental retardation significant social incompetency due to developmental limitations of general intelligence.

metabolism the rate at which body cells exchange nutrients, gases, and waste material.

metaphor a figure of speech suggesting an analogy between things normally seen as different: e.g., "The ship *plows* the waves."

methylphenidate a drug commonly referred to as Ritalin, frequently given to hyperactive children.

modality referring to the mode or form of learning or communication (auditory, visual, kinesthetic).

morpheme the smallest meaningful language units (sounds, words).

morphology the study of meaningful verbal concepts and the rules for creating words.

multisensory the use of several senses together in learning or problem solving.

myelination the growth of a soft, fatty, white substance protecting certain nerve fibers.

neuropsychological brain processes underlying patterns of behavior.

neuropsychological education special training that attempts to improve brain functioning and operation.

neuropsychological processing the internal neurological and psychological responses and operations involved in associating and responding to external stimuli and information.

nystagmus uncoordinated rapid eye movements.

occipital lobe the back portion of each hemisphere concerned with visual integration.

ocular pursuit following a moving target with the eyes. Requires convergence and coordinated tracking.

optic chiasma the place where nerve impulses from each eye are transmitted to opposite sides of the brain.

parietal lobe the middle portion of each cerebral hemisphere. Largely concerned with kinesthetic-tactile-motor integration functions.

patterning the direct attempt to impose complex bodily patterns or movements by external manipulation or exercise of those body parts.

phoneme the smallest sound unit in a language.

phonics a method of teaching reading, pronunciation, and spelling based on the interpretation of speech sounds.

proprioceptive relating to sensory excitations originating within the individual from kinesthetic-muscular movements.

psychoeducational specific educational learning tasks and conditions that change behavior.

psycholinguistics the mental operations involved in the understanding and use of language.

reading a linguistic process of decoding and attributing meaning to speech that has been written down in the form of graphic symbols.

reinforcement the strengthening of acquired behavior through systematic rewards and encouragement.

reticular system neural fibers extending in a midbrain network responsible for controlling arousal and excitation.

retina the rear lining of the eyeball, which receives light stimuli.

saccade short, quickly-focused eye movements.

self-concept how a person thinks and feels about him or herself as a person.

semantics the study of word meanings and human reactions to words beyond their basic meanings.

significance a term referring to high importance of statistical validity or verification.

stereoreader an instrument for developing laterality in reading and visual-motor exercises.

sterognosis the identification and knowledge of objects through the sense of touch.

strephosymbolia twisting or reversing letter symbols in reading or perception.

supination placing or turning on the backside (for example, turning the palms of the hands up).

syllable a segment of speech expressed in sounds or written form.

synapse the region of contact between two nerve cells across which an electrochemical impulse passes.

syntax sentence structure.

tachistoscope an instrument that exposes words or symbols for a brief period of time.

task analysis evaluation of the specific learning task, item, or problem.

temporal lobe the outer and underside of each hemisphere largely concerned with auditory integration.

thalamus part of the midbrain through which sensory impulses pass to the cerebral cortex.

vestibular referring to the ear cavity and labyrinth largely concerned with stability and balance.

visual pertaining to sight.

word blindness loss of ability to recognize the meanings of printed or written words.

References

Chapter One

Bond, G., and Tinker, M. *Reading Difficulties: Their Diagnosis and Correction*. 3d ed. Englewood Cliffs, N.J.: Prentice-Hall, 1973.

Chall, J. *Learning to Read: The Great Debate*. New York: McGraw-Hill, 1967.

Christensen, A. *Luria's Neuropsychological Investigation*. New York: John Wiley/Spectrum, 1975.

Critchley, M. *The Dyslexic Child*. London: William Heinemann Medical Books, 1970.

Dale, P. *Language Development: Structure and Function*. Hinsdale, Ill.: Dryden Press, 1972.

de Hirsch, K. "Clinical Spectrum of Reading and Disabilities: Diagnosis and Treatment." *Bulletin of the New York Academy of Medicine* 44(1968): 470-77.

Drew, A. "A Neurological Appraisal of Familial Congenital Word Blindness. *Brain* 79(1956):440-60.

Durrell, D. *Improvement of Basic Reading Abilities*. New York: World Book Co., 1940.

Goldberg, H., and Schiffman, G. *Dyslexia*. New York: Grune and Stratton, 1972.

Hepworth, T. *Dyslexia—The Problem of Reading Retardation*. Sydney, Australia: Angus and Robertson, 1971.

Hinshelwood, J. *Congenital Word-Blindness*. London: Lewis, 1917.

Johnson, D., and Myklebust, H. *Learning Disabilities: Educational Principles and Practices*. New York: Grune and Stratton, 1967.

Kasen, E. *The Syndrome of Specific Dyslexia*. Baltimore: University Park Press, 1972.

McGrady, H., Jr. "Language Pathology and Learning Disabilities." In *Progress in Learning Disabilities*, vol. 1, edited by H. Myklebust, pp. 199-233. New York: Grune and Stratton, 1968.

Myklebust, H., ed. *Progress in Learning Disabilities*, vol. 1. New York: Grune and Stratton, 1968.

Myklebust, H., and Johnson, D. "Dyslexia in Children." *Exceptional Children* 29(1962): 14-25.

Orton, S. *Reading, Writing, and Speech Problems in Children*. 1937. Reprint. New York: W. W. Norton, 1964.

———. "Specific Reading Disability: Strephosymbolia." *Journal of the American Medical Association* 90(1928):1095-99.

Rosinski, R. *The Development of Visual Perception*. Santa Monica, Calif.: Goodyear Publishing Co., 1977.

U.S., Department of Health, Education and Welfare, Office of Education. *Problems of Dyslexia and Related Disorders*, Research Conference Report, Washington, D.C., July 12, 1967.

Valett, R. *Developing Cognitive Abilities: Teaching Children to Think*. St. Louis: C. V. Mosby, 1978.

Chapter Two

Ackerman, P.; Peters, J.; and Dykman, R. "Children with Learning Disabilities: WISC Profiles." *Journal of Learning Disabilities* 4(1971)150-66.

Ames, L. "Learning Disabilities: The Developmental Point of View." In *Progress in Learning Disabilities,* vol. 1, edited by H. Myklebust, pp. 39-74. New York: Grune and Stratton, 1968.

Bakker, D. "Ear-Asymmetry with Monaural Stimulation." *Psychonomic Science* 12 (1968):62.

Birch, H., and Belmont, L. "Auditory-Visual Integration in Normal and Retarded Readers." *American Journal of Orthopsychiatry* 34(1964):852-61.

Christensen, A. *Luria's Neuropsychological Investigation.* New York: John Wiley/Spectrum, 1975.

Corkin, S. "Serial-ordering Deficits in Inferior Readers." *Neuropsychologia* 12(1974):347-54.

Doehring, D. *Patterns of Impairment in Specific Reading Disability—A Neuropsychological Investigation.* Bloomington, Ind.: Indiana University Press, 1968.

Drew, A. "A Neurological Appraisal of Familial Cogenital Word Blindness." *Brain* 79(1956):440-60.

Dykman, R.; Ackerman, P.; Clements, S.; and Peters, J. "Specific Learning Disabilities: An Attentional Deficit Syndrome." In *Progress in Learning Disabilities,* vol. 2, edited by H. Myklebust, pp. 56-93. New York: Grune and Stratton, 1971.

Dykstra, R., and Tinney, R. "Sex Differences in Reading Readiness: First Grade Achievement and Second Grade Achievement." In *Reading and Realism,* edited by J. Figurel, pp. 623-28. Newark, Del.: International Reading Association, 1969.

Ekstrand, L. "Social and Individual Frame Factors in L2 Learning: Comparative Aspects." Paper presented at the First Scandinavian Conference on Bilingualism, Helsinki, Finland, September 27-30, 1976.

Frank J., and Levinson. H. "Dysmetric Dyslexia and Dyspraxia." *Academic Therapy Quarterly* 11(1975-76):133-42.

————. "Compensatory Mechanisms in Cerebellar-Vestibular Dysfunction, Dysmetric Dyslexia, and Dyspraxia." *Academic Therapy Quarterly* 12(1976):5-27.

Goins, J. *Visual Perception Abilities and Early Reading Progress,* Supplemental Education Monograph no. 87. Chicago: University of Chicago Press, 1958.

Goldstein, K. *Language and Language Disturbances.* New York: Grune and Stratton, 1948.

Gray, C. *Deficiencies in Reading Ability, Their Diagnosis and Remedies.* Boston: Health, 1922.

Hughes, J. "Biochemical and Electroencephalographic Correlates of Learning Disabilities." In *The Neuropsychology of Learning Disorders,* edited by R. Knights and D. Bakker, pp. 53-69. Baltimore: University Park Press, 1976.

Ilg, F., and Ames, L. *School Readiness.* New York: Harper & Row, 1965.

Jastak, J., and Jastak, S. *Wide Range Achievement Test Manual.* Wilmington, Del.: Guidance Associates, 1976.

Kass, C. "Some Psychological Correlates of Severe Reading Disability (Dyslexia)." Doctoral dissertation, University of Illinois, 1962.

Katz, P., and Deutsch, M. "Relation of Auditory-Visual Shifting to Reading Achievement." *Perceptual and Motor Skills* 17 (1963):327-32.

Lawson, L., Jr. "Ophthalmological Factors in Learning Disabilities." In *Progress in Learning Disabilities,* vol. 1, edited by H. Myklebust, pp. 147-81. New York: Grune and Stratton, 1968.

Leong, C. "Lateralization in Severely Disabled Readers in Relation to Functional Cerebral Development and Synthesis of Information." In *The Neuropsychology of Learning Disorders,* edited by R. Knights and D. Bakker, pp. 221-31. Baltimore: University Park Press, 1976.

Levine, M. "Physiological Responses in Intra-sensory and Intersensory Integration of Auditory and Visual Signals by Normal and Deficit Readers," In *The Neuropsychology of Learning Disorders,* edited by R. Knights and D. Bakker, pp. 99–110. Baltimore: University Park Press, 1976.

Linksz, A. *On Writing, Reading, and Dyslexia.* New York: Grune and Stratton, 1973.

Luria, A. *Restoration of Function after Brain Injury.* New York: Macmillan/Pergamon, 1963.

_____. *Higher Cortical Functions in Man.* New York: Basic Books, 1966.

_____. *The Working Brain: An Introduction to Neuropsychology.* New York: Basic Books, 1973.

MacBurney, N., and Dunn, H. "Handedness, Footedness, Eyedness: A Prospective Study with Special Reference to the Development of Speech and Language Skills. In *The Neuropsychology of Learning Disorders,* edited by R. Knights and D. Bakker, pp. 139–48. Baltimore: University Park Press, 1976.

Mariam, S. "A Comparative Study of the Reading Disability in Neurologically Organized and Neurologically Disorganized Fifth Grade Children." In *Neurological Organization and Reading,* edited by C. Delacato, pp. 75–108. Springfield, Ill.: Charles C. Thomas, 1966.

Owen, F.; Adams, P.; Forrest, T.; Stolz, L.; and Fisher, S. "Learning Disorders in Children: Sibling Studies." *Monographs of the Society for Research in Child Development* 36 (Serial no. 144), 1971.

Prechtl, H. "Reading Difficulties as a Neurological Problem in Childhood." In *Reading Disability,* edited by J. Money. Baltimore: Johns Hopkins Press, 1962.

Rourke, B. "Brain-Behavior Relationships in Children with Learning Disabilities: A Research Program." *American Psychologist* 30(1975):911–19.

Satz, P. "Cerebral Dominance and Reading Disability: An Old Problem Revisited." In *The Neuropsychology of Learning Dis-orders,* edited by R. Knights and D. Bakker, pp. 273–94. Baltimore: University Park Press, 1976.

Satz, P., and Van Nostrand, G. "Developmental Dyslexia: An Evaluation of a Theory." In *The Disabled Learner: Early Detection and Intervention,* edited by P. Satz and J. Ross, pp. 121–48. Rotterdam: Rotterdam University Press, 1973.

Sheer, D. "Biofeedback Training of 40Hz EEG and Behavior." In *Behavior and Brain Electrical Activity,* edited by N. Burch and H. Altschuler. New York: Plenum Press, 1975.

Tallal, P. "Auditory Perceptual Factors in Language and Learning Disabilities." In *The Neuropsychology of Learning Disorders,* edited by R. Knights and D. Bakker, pp. 315–25. Baltimore: University Park Press, 1976.

Taylor, E. *The Fundamental Reading Skill.* Springfield, Ill.: Charles C. Thomas, 1966.

Van Duyne, H., and Bakker, D. "The Development of Ear-Asymmetry Related to Coding Processes in Memory in Children." Paper presented at the fourth annual meeting of the International Neuropsychological Society, Toronto, 1976.

Witelson, S. "Abnormal Right Hemisphere Specialization in Developmental Dyslexia." In *The Neuropsychology of Learning Disorders,* edited by R. Knights and D. Bakker, pp. 233–55. Baltimore: University Park Press, 1976.

Zigmond, N. "Intrasensory and Intersensory Processes in Normal and Dyslexic Children." Doctoral dissertation, Northwestern University, 1966.

Chapter Three

Altman, J., and Dos, G. "Behavioral Manipulation and Protein Metabolism of the Brain: Effects of Motor Exercise on the Utilization of Leucine-H^3." *Physiological Behavior* 1(1966):105–8.

Ayres, A. "Improving Academic Scores through Sensory Integration." *Journal of Learning Disabilities* 5(1972):338–43.

_____.*Sensory Integration and Learning Disorders.* Los Angeles: Western Psychological Services, 1972a.

Bogen, J.; Fisher, E.; and Vogel, P. "Cerebral Commisurotomy: A Second Case Report." *Journal of the American Medical Association* 194(1965):1328-29.

Diamond, M; Law, F.; Rhodes, H.; Lindner, B.; Rosenzweig, M.; Krech, D.; and Bennett, E. "Increases in Cortical Depth and Glia Numbers in Rats Subjected to Enriched Environment." *Journal of Comparative Neurology* 128(1966):117-25.

Eccles, J. *The Understanding of the Brain.* New York: McGraw-Hill, 1972.

Eccles, J.; Ito, M.; and Szentagothai, J. *The Cerebellum as a Neuronal Machine.* New York: Springer-Verlag, 1967.

Fishbein, H. *Evolution, Development and Children's Learning.* Santa Monica, Calif.: Goodyear Publishing Co., 1976.

Galin, D., and Ornstein, R. "Lateral Specialization of the Cognitive Mode: An EEG Study." *Psychophysiology* 9(1972):412-18.

Gazzangia, M. "The Split Brain in Man." *Scientific American* 217(1967):24-29.

Greisheimer, E. *Physiology and Anatomy.* Philadelphia: J. B. Lippincott, 1945.

Hebb, D. *The Organization of Behavior: A Neuropsychological Theory.* New York: John Wiley, 1949.

Hebb, D.; Lambert, W.; and Tucker, G. "A DMZ in the Language War." *Psychology Today,* April 1973, pp. 55-62.

Hydén, H., and Lange, P. "Protein Synthesis in the Hippocampal Pyramidal Cells of Rats During a Behavioral Test." *Science* 159 (1970):1370-73.

Ingvar, D., and Schwartz, M. "Brain Blood Flow Patterns Induced in the Dominant Hemisphere by Speech and Reading." *Brain* 97(1974):273-88.

Krech, D.; Rosenzweig, M.; and Bennett, E. "Environmental Impoverishment, Social Isolation, and Changes in Brain Chemistry and Anatomy." *Physiology and Behavior* 1 (1966):99-104.

_____."Relations between Brain Chemistry and Problem-Solving among Rats Raised in Enriched and Impoverished Environments." *Journal of Physiological Psychology* 55 (1962):801-7.

Levin, J., and Allen, V., eds. *Cognitive Learning in Children.* New York: Academic Press, 1976.

Levy, J. "Expressive Language in the Surgically Separated Minor Hemisphere." *Cortex* 47(1972):49-58.

_____."Possible Basis for the Evolution of Lateral Specialization in the Human Brain." *Nature* 224(1967):614-15.

Luria, A. *The Working Brain: An Introduction to Neuropsychology.* New York: Basic Books, 1973.

Meichenbaum, D. "Cognitive-Functional Approach to Cognitive Factors as Determinants of Learning Disabilities." In *The Neuropsychology of Learning Disorders,* edited by R. Knights and D. Bakker, pp. 423-41. Baltimore: University Park Press, 1976.

Piaget, J. *The Origins of Intelligence in Children.* New York: W. W. Norton, 1952.

Pines, M. "Can the Brain Renew Itself?" *Psychology* 1(1977):16-19.

Sperry, R. "Hemispheric Disconnection and Unity in Conscious Awareness." *American Psychologist* 23(1968):723-33.

Valett, R. *Developing Cognitive Abilities: Teaching Children to Think.* St. Louis: C. V. Mosby, 1978.

Whittrock, M. "The Generative Process of Memory." *UCLA Educator* 17(1975):33-34.

Chapter Four

Ammon, P., and Ammon, M. "Effects of Training Black Preschool Children in Vocabulary versus Sentence Construction." *Journal of Educational Psychology* 62(1971): 421-26.

Arena, J. *Building Spelling Skills in Dyslexic Children.* San Rafael, Calif.: Academic Therapy Publications, 1968.

Arnold, L.; Huestis, R.; Wemmer, D.; and

Smeltzer, D. "Differential Effect of Amphetamine Optical Isomers on Bender Gestalt Performance of the Minimally Brain Dysfunctioned." *Journal of Learning Disabilities* 11(1978):127–32.

Bannatyne, A. "Diagnostic and Remedial Techniques for Use with Dyslexic Children." *Academic Therapy Quarterly* 3(1968): 213–33.

Bellugi-Klima, U., and Hass, W. "Syntactical Structures for Modeling in Preschool Language Training." In *Promising Practices in Language Training in Early Childhood Education,* edited by C. Lavatelli. Urbana, Ill.: University of Illinois Press, ERIC Clearinghouse on Early Childhood Education, 1968.

Bereiter, C., and Engelmann, S. *Teaching Disadvantaged Children in the Preschool.* Englewood Cliffs, N.J.: Prentice-Hall, 1966.

Bernstein, N. "The Effect of Training in the Cognitive Uses of Language on the Attainment and Retention of Double Classification Concepts by Kindergarten Children." Doctoral dissertation, New York University, 1969.

Blank, M., and Solomon, F. "A Tutorial Language Program to Develop Abstract Thinking in Socially Disadvantaged Preschool Children." *Child Development* 39(1968): 379–90.

Bloom, L., and Lahey, M. *Language Development and Language Disorders.* New York: John Wiley, 1978.

Boehm, A. *Boehm Test of Basic Concepts.* New York: The Psychological Corp., 1967.

Brainerd, C. "Training and Transfer of Transitivity, Conservation, and Class Inclusion of Length." *Child Development* 45(1974): 324–34.

Bricker, W., and Bricker, D. "An Early Language Training Strategy." In *Language Perspectives Acquisition, Retardation, and Intervention,* edited by P. Schiefelbusch and L. Loyd, pp. 429–68. Baltimore: University Park Press, 1974.

Bruner, J. "Play Is Serious Business." *Psychology Today,* January 1975, pp. 81–83.

Caldwell, E., and Hall, V. "The Influence of Concept Training on Letter Discrimination." *Child Development* 40(1969):63–71.

Childs, S., ed. *Education and Specific Language Disability: The Papers of Anna Gillingham.* Towson, Md.: The Orton Society, 1968.

Chomsky, N. *Language and Mind.* New York: Harcourt Brace Jovanovich, 1972.

Conger, J.; Kagan, J.; and Mussen, P. *Child Development and Personality.* New York: Harper & Row, 1969.

Courtright, J., and Courtright, I. "Imitative Modeling as a Theoretical Base for Instructing Language Disordered Children." *Journal of Speech and Hearing Research* 19(1976): 655–63.

Dale, P. *Language Development: Structure and Function.* Hinsdale, Ill.; Dryden Press, 1972.

Darnell, L., and Molineux, M. *Suggested Activities: Language Development Program for the Mentally Retarded.* Springfield, Ill.: Department of Mental Health, H. Douglas Singer Zone Center, 1972.

Denckla, M. "The Neurological Basis of Reading Disability." In *Reading Disability.* 3d rev. ed., edited by F. Roswell and G. Natchez. New York: Basic Books, 1977.

De Pauw, K. "Enhancing the Sensory Integration of Aphasic Students." *Journal of Learning Disabilities* 11(1978):142–46.

DeVilliers, J., and Naughton, J. "Teaching a Symbol Language to Autistic Children." *Journal of Consulting and Clinical Psychology* 42(1974):111–17.

Eisenson, J., and Ingram, D. "Childhood Aphasia: An Updated Concept Based on Recent Research." *Acta Symbolica* 3(1972): 108–16.

Enstrom, E., and Enstrom, D. "Imprint Handwriting: Preventing and Solving Reversal Problems." *Elementary English* 31(1969): 759–64.

Farr, R. *Reading: What Can Be Measured?* Newark, Del.: International Reading Association, 1969.

Gardner, H. "The Forgotten Lesson of Monsieur C." *Psychology Today* August 1973, pp. 63–68.

Geschwind, N. "Language and the Brain." *Scientific American* 226(1972):76–86.

Gillingham, A., and Stillman, B. *Remedial Training for Children with Specific Language Disability in Reading, Spelling, and Penmanship.* 6th ed. Cambridge, Mass.: Educators Publishing Service, 1960.

Giordano, G. "Convergent Research on Language and Teaching Reading." *Exceptional Children* 44(1978):604–10.

Gomez, M. *Neurological Approach to Specific Language Disability.* Towson, Md.: The Orton Society, 1971.

Griffiths, A. "WISC as a Diagnostic-Remedial Tool for Dyslexia." *Academic Therapy Quarterly* 12(1977):401–9.

Grinnell, M.; Detamore, K.; and Lippke, B. "Sign It Successful: Manual English Encourages Expressive Communication." *Teaching Exceptional Children* 42(1976): 123–24.

Hallenbeck, P. "Remediating with Comic Strips." *Journal of Learning Disabilities* 9 (1976):11–12.

Heber, R. "Sociocultural Mental Retardation: A Longitudinal Study." Madison, Wis.: University of Wisconsin, Rehabilitation Research and Training Center in Mental Retardation. Paper presented at the Vermont conference on the primary prevention of psychopathology, June 1976.

Heber, R.; Garber, H.; Harrington, S.; Hoffman, C.; and Falender, C. "Rehabilitation of Families at Risk for Mental Retardation: Progress Report." Madison, Wis.: University of Wisconsin, Rehabilitation Research and Training Center in Mental Retardation, 1972.

Jensen, A. "How Much Can We Boost IQ and Scholastic Achievement?" *Harvard Educational Review* 39(1969):1–123.

Kaplan-Fitzgerald, K. *Reach Me Teach Me.* San Rafael, Calif.: Academic Therapy Publications, 1977.

Keeney, H., and Keeney, V. *Dyslexia: Diagnosis and Treatment of Reading Disorders.* St. Louis: C. V. Mosby, 1966.

Kirk, S.; Kliebhan, S.; and Lerner, J. *Teaching Reading to Slow and Disabled Learners.* Boston: Houghton Mifflin, 1978.

Klaus, R., and Gray, S. "The Early Training Project for Disadvantaged Children: A Report after Five Years." *Monographs of the Society for Research in Child Development* 33(1968):4.

Kohl, H. *Language and Education of the Deaf.* Policy Study 1. New York: Center for Urban Education, 1966.

Lahey, M., ed. *Readings in Childhood Language Disorders.* New York: John Wiley, 1978.

Larsen, G. "Developmental Study of the Relation between Conservation and Sharing Behavior." *Child Development* 40(1974):850.

Laurita, R. "Reversals: A Response to Frustrations?" *The Reading Teacher* 25(1971): 45–52.

Lavatelli, C. *Piaget's Theory Applied to an Early Childhood Curriculum.* Boston: Center for Media Development, 1970.

Lovaas, O.; Berberich, J.; Perloff, B.; and Schaeffer, B. "Acquisition of Imitative Speech in Schizophrenic Children." *Science* 151(1966):705–7.

Masland, R. *Brain Mechanisms Underlying the Language Function.* Towson, Md.: The Orton Society, 1967.

Milner, E. "A Study of the Relationship between Reading Readiness in Grade One School Children and Patterns of Parent-Child Interaction." *Child Development* 22(1951):95–112.

Monaco, L., and Zaslow, E. *Hey, I Got Sump'n to Tell You, an' It Cool: A Class for Children with Severe Language Disabilities.* Rockville, Md.: Montgomery County Public Schools Board of Education, 1972.

Myklebust, H. *Development and Disorders of Written Language,* vol. 1. New York: Grune and Stratton, 1965.

Nemac, R. "Effects of Controlled Background Interference on Test Performance of Right and Left Hemiplegics." *Journal of Consulting and Clinical Psychology* 46(1978): 294–97.

Orton, S. *Reading, Writing, and Speech Problems in Children.* 1937. Reprint. New York: W. W. Norton, 1964.

Osgood, C. *Approaches to the Study of Aphasia.* Urbana, Ill.: University of Illinois Press, 1963.

Piaget, J. *Play, Dreams, and Imitation in Childhood.* New York: W. W. Norton, 1951.

Piaget, J., and Inhelder, B. *The Psychology of the Child.* New York: Basic Books, 1969.

Reed, H., Jr.; Reitan, R.; and Kløve, H. "Influence of Cerebral Lesions on Psychological Test Performance of Older Children." *Journal of Consulting Psychology* 29(1965):247–51.

Sabatino, D. "Identifying Neurologically Impaired Children through a Test of Auditory Perception." *Journal of Consulting and Clinical Psychology* 33(1969):184–88.

Satz, P. "Cerebral Dominance and Reading Disability: An Old Problem Revisited." In *The Neuropsychology of Learning Disorders,* edited by R. Knights and D. Bakker, pp. 273–94. Baltimore: University Park Press, 1976.

Schiefelbusch, R.; Copeland, R.; and Smith, J. *Language and Mental Retardation.* New York: Holt, Rinehart, and Winston, 1967.

Schuell, H. *Aphasia Theory and Therapy.* Baltimore: University Park Press, 1974.

Searls, E. *How to Use WISC Scores in Reading Diagnosis.* Newark, Del.: International Reading Association, 1975.

Snyder, L.; Lovitt, T.; and Smith, J. "Language Training for the Severely Retarded: Five Years of Behavior Analysis Research." *Exceptional Children* 41(1975):1–16.

Taylor, A.; Thurlow, M.; and Turnure, J. "Vocabulary Development of Educable Retarded Children." *Exceptional Children* 43(1977):444–49.

Taylor, E. "Jimmy: Extra Pyramidal Lesion, Athetosis, Dysarthria, Auditory Defect." In *Psychological Appraisal of Children with Cerebral Defects,* pp. 136–81. Cambridge, Mass.: Harvard University Press, 1961.

Thompson, L. "Language Disabilities in Men of Eminence." *Journal of Learning Disabilities* 4(1971):39–44.

U.S., Department of Health, Education and Welfare, Office of Education. *Assistance to States for Education of Handicapped Children: Procedures for Evaluating Specific Learning Disabilities.* Federal Register 42 (250), 1977.

Valett, R. *The Remediation of Learning Disabilities.* 2d ed. Belmont, Calif.: Fearon Pitman, 1974.

———. *Developing Cognitive Abilities: Teaching Children to Think.* St. Louis: C. V. Mosby, 1978.

Vellutino, F. "Alternative Conceptualization of Dyslexia: Evidence in Support of a Verbal-Deficit Hypothesis." *Harvard Educational Review* 47(1977):334–49.

Wood, N. *Delayed Speech and Language Development.* Englewood Cliffs, N.J.: Prentice-Hall, 1964.

Chapter 5

Anatasi, A. *Psychological Testing.* 4th ed. New York: Macmillan, 1976.

Ayres, A. *Sensory Integration and Learning Disorders.* Los Angeles: Western Psychological Services, 1973.

———. "Learning Disabilities and the Vestibular System." *Journal of Learning Disabilities* 11(1978):30–41.

Birch, H., and Belmont, L. "Auditory-Visual Integration, Intelligence, and Reading Ability in School Children." *Perceptual and Motor Skills* 20(1965):295–305.

Bond, G., and Tinker, M. *Reading Difficulties: Their Diagnosis and Correction.* New York: Appleton-Century-Crofts, 1957.

Brueckner, L., and Bond, G. *The Diagnosis and Treatment of Learning Difficulties.* New

York: Appleton-Century-Crofts, 1955.

Christensen, A. *Luria's Neuropsychological Investigation.* New York: John Wiley/Spectrum, 1975.

Dunn, L. *Exceptional Children in the Schools.* New York: Holt, Rinehart, and Winston, 1963.

Ferinden, W., and Jacobson, S. *Educational Interpretation of the Wechsler Intelligence Scale for Children.* Linden, N.J.: Remediation Associates, 1969.

Geschwind, N. "The Anatomy of Acquired Disorders in Reading." In *Reading Disability: Progress and Research Needs in Dyslexia,* edited by J. Money, pp. 115–29. Baltimore: Johns Hopkins Press, 1962.

Glasser, A., and Zimmerman, I. *Clinical Interpretation of the Wechsler Intelligence Scale for Children.* New York: Grune and Stratton, 1967.

Jastak, J., and Jastak, S. *Wide Range Achievement Test Manual.* Wilmington, Del.: Guidance Associates, 1976.

Jordan, D. *Dyslexia in the Classroom.* Columbus, Ohio: Charles E. Merrill, 1972.

Kirk, S. *Educating Exceptional Children.* Boston: Houghton Mifflin, 1962.

Mutti, M.; Sterling, H.; Spalding, N.; and Crawford, C. *Quick Neurological Screening Test Manual.* San Rafael, Calif.: Academic Therapy Publications, 1974.

Powell, H., and Chansky, N. "The Evaluation of Academic Disabilities." In *School Psychological Services,* edited by J. Magary, pp. 523–52. Englewood Cliffs, N.J.: Prentice-Hall, 1967.

Rabinovitch, R. "Reading and Learning Disabilities." In *American Handbook of Psychiatry.* vol. 1, edited by S. Arieti, pp. 857–69. New York: Basic Books, 1959.

Satz, P. and Friel, J. "Some Predictive Antecedents of Specific Reading Disability: A Preliminary Two-Year Follow-up. *Journal of Learning Disabilities* 7(1974):48–55.

Searls, E. *How to Use WISC Scores in Reading Diagnosis.* Newark, Del.: International Reading Association, 1975.

Spache, G. *Investigating the Issues of Reading Disabilities.* Boston: Allyn and Bacon, 1976.

Thomas, G., and Cresimbeni, J. *Guiding the Gifted Child.* New York: Random House, 1966.

Valett, R. *Programming Learning Disabilities.* Belmont, Calif.: Fearon Pitman, 1969.

_____. *Learning Disabilities: Diagnostic-Prescriptive Instruments.* Belmont, Calif.: Fearon Pitman, 1973.

_____. *Developing Cognitive Abilities: Teaching Children to Think.* St. Louis: C. V. Mosby, 1978.

Wechsler, D. *Manual for the WISC-R.* New York: The Psychological Corporation, 1974.

Chapter Six

Ayres, A. "Improving Academic Scores through Sensory Integration." *Journal of Learning Disabilities* 5(1972):338–43.

_____. *Sensory Integration and Learning Disorders.* Los Angeles: Western Psychological Services, 1972.

Cratty, B. *Educational Implications of Movement Experiences.* Seattle, Wash.: Special Child Publications, 1970.

_____. *Active Learning: Games to Enhance Academic Abilities.* Englewood Cliffs, N.J.: Prentice-Hall, 1971.

_____. *Intelligence in Action.* Englewood Cliffs, N.J.: Prentice-Hall, 1973.

Delacato, C., ed. *Neurological Organization and Reading.* Springfield, Ill.: Charles C. Thomas, 1966.

Doman, R.; Spitz, E.; Zucman, E.; Delacato, C.; and Doman, G. "Children with Severe Brain Injuries: Neurological Organization in Terms of Mobility." *Journal of the American Medical Association* 174(1960):257–62.

Faustman, M. "Some Effects of Perception Training in Kindergarten on First Grade Success in Reading." In *Perception and Reading,* edited by H. Smith, pp. 99–101. Newark, Del.: International Reading Association, 1968.

Heber, R.; Garber, H.; Harrington, S.; Hoffman, C.; and Falender, C. "Rehabilitation of Families at Risk for Mental Retardation: Progress Report." Madison, Wis.: University of Wisconsin, Rehabilitation Research and Training Center in Mental Retardation, 1972.

LeWinn, E. *Human Neurological Organization.* Springfield, Ill.: Charles C. Thomas, 1969.

Luria, A. *Restoration of Function after Brain Injury.* New York: Macmillan/Pergamon, 1963.

Mariam, S. "A Comparative Study of the Reading Disability in Neurologically Organized and Neurologically Disorganized Fifth Grade Children." In *Neurological Organization and Reading,* edited by C. Delacato, pp. 75–108. Springfield, Ill.: Charles C. Thomas, 1966.

Miracle, B. "The Linguistic Effects of Neuropsychological Techniques in Treating a Selected Group of Retarded Readers." In *Neurological Organization and Reading,* edited by C. Delacato, pp. 156–79. Springfield, Ill.: Charles C. Thomas, 1966.

Montessori, M. *The Montessori Method.* Rev. ed. New York: Schocken Books, 1964.

Painter, G. "The Effect of Rhythmic and Sensory Motor Activity Programs on Perceptual Motor Spatial Abilities of Kindergarten Children." *Exceptional Children* 33(1966):113–16.

Semans, S. "Physical Therapy for Motor Disorders Resulting from Brain Damage." *Rehabilitation Literature* 20(1959):99–110.

Valett, R. *Learning Disabilities: Diagnostic-Prescriptive Instruments.* Belmont, Calif.: Fearon Pitman, 1973.

_____. *The Remediation of Learning Disabilities.* 2d ed. Belmont, Calif.: Fearon Pitman, 1974.

Chapter Seven

Bakker, D. "Perceptual Asymmetries and Reading Proficiency." In *Toward Theories of Cognitive Development,* edited by M. Bortner. New York: Brunner-Mazel, 1977.

Behrmann, P. *Activities for Developing Visual Perception.* San Rafael, Calif.: Academic Therapy Publications, 1970.

Boucher, S. "The Effects of Memory Training on Reading Achievement." Master's thesis, California State University, Fresno, 1976.

Denckla, M. "The Neurological Basis of Reading Disability." In *Reading Disability,* edited by F. Roswell and G. Natchez, pp. 25–47. New York: Basic Books, 1977.

DeVilliers, J., and Naughton, J. "Teaching a Symbol Language to Autistic Children." *Journal of Consulting and Clinical Psychology* 42(1974):111–17.

Dolch, E. *Teaching Pirmary Reading.* Champaign, Ill.: Garrard Publishing Company, 1960.

Dunn, L. "The Efficacy of the Initial Teaching Alphabet and the Peabody Language Development Kit with Disadvantaged Children in the Primary Grades: An Interim Report." *IMRID Paper.* Peabody College, Nashville, Tenn., 1967.

Gates, A. "Psychology of Reading and Spelling with Special Reference to Disability." *Contributions to Education.* no. 129. New York: Bureau of Publication, Teachers College, Columbia University, 1922.

Gattegno, C. *Words in Color: A New Method of Teaching the Reading and Writing of English.* New York: Xerox Corporation, 1963.

Goins, J. *Visual Perception Abilities and Early Reading Progress.* Supplemental Education Monograph no. 87. Chicago: University of Chicago Press, 1958.

Gray, C. *Deficiencies in Reading Ability, Their Diagnosis and Remedies.* Boston: Health, 1922.

Groff, P. " 'Sight' Words and the Disabled Reader." *Academic Therapy Quarterly* 10 (1974):101–7.

Halliwell, J., and Solan, H. "The Effects of a Supplemental Perceptual Training Program on Reading Achievement." *Exceptional Children* 38(1972):613–22.

Kaluger, G., and Kolson, C. *Reading and Learning Disabilities.* Columbus, Ohio: Charles E. Merrill, 1969.

Kass, C. "Some Psychological Correlates of Severe Reading Disability (Dyslexia)." Doctoral dissertation, University of Illinois, 1962.

Leisman, G. "The Role of Visual Processes in Attention and Its Disorders." In *Basic Visual Processes and Learning Disability,* edited by G. Leisman. Springfield, Ill.: Charles C. Thomas, 1975.

Lundberg, T. "Aspects of Cognitive Psychology as Related to Beginning Reading." *Skolepsykologi* (Denmark) 14(1977):165–89.

Lyle, J., and Goyen, J. "Visual Recognition, Developmental Lag, and Strephosymbolia in Reading Retardation." *Journal of Abnormal Psychology* 73(1968):25–29.

Mackworth, J. "Some Models of the Reading Process: Learners and Skilled Readers." In *Children with Learning Problems,* edited by S. Sapir and A. Nitzburg, pp. 485–516. New York: Brunner-Mazel, 1973.

Miller, L., and Turner, S. "Development of Hemifield Differences in Word Recognition." *Journal of Educational Psychology* 65(1973):172–76.

Morrison, F.; Giordani, B.; and Nagy, J. "Reading Disability: An Information-Processing Analysis." *Science* 196(1977):77–79.

Moyer, S., and Newcomer, P. "Reversals in Reading: Diagnosis and Remediation." *Exceptional Children* 43(1977):424–30.

Muehl, S., and King, E. "Recent Research in Visual Discrimination: Significance for Beginning Reading." In *Vistas for Reading,* edited by J. Figurel, pp. 434–39. Newark, Del.: International Reading Association, 1967.

Oliphant, G. *A Study of Factors Involved in Early Identification of Specific Language Disability.* Towson, Md.: The Orton Society, 1969.

Rizzo, N. "Studies in Visual and Auditory Memory Span with Special Reference to Reading Disability." *Journal of Experimental Education* 8(1939):208–44.

Roswell, F., and Natchez, G., eds. *Reading Disability.* 3d rev. ed. New York: Basic Books, 1977.

Rudel, R.; Denckla, M.; and Spalten, E. "Paired Associative Learning of Morse Code and Braille Letter Names by Dyslexic and Normal Children." *Cortex* 12(1976):61–70.

Sells, S., and Fixott, R. "Evaluation of Research on Effects of Visual Training in Visual Functions." *American Journal of Ophthalmology* 44(1957):230.

Spache, G. "A Summary of Apparently Successful Perceptual Training Programs." Table 16-2 in *Investigating the Issues in Reading Disabilities,* pp. 417–18. Boston: Allyn and Bacon, 1976.

Swanson, W. "Visually Related Learning Disorders." Special reprint, *Journal of the California Optometric Association.* December–January 1971–72.

Trela, T. *Fourteen Remedial Reading Methods.* Belmont, Calif.: Fearon Pitman, 1968.

Venezky, R. "Research on Reading Processes: A Historical Perspective." *American Psychologist* 32(1977):339–45.

Wiig, E., and Semel, E. *Language Disabilities in Children and Adolescents.* Columbus, Ohio: Charles E. Merrill, 1976.

Witelson, S. "Abnormal Right Hemisphere Specialization in Developmental Dyslexia." In *The Neuropsychology of Learning Disorders,* edited by R. Knights and D. Bakker, pp. 233–55. Baltimore: University Park Press, 1976.

Woodcock, R. "Rebus as a Medium in Beginning Reading Instruction." *IMRID Paper,* no. 4, Peabody College, Nashville, Tenn., 1968.

Chapter Eight

American Academy of Ophthalmology and Otolaryngology. *A Guide to the Care of*

Adults with Hearing Loss. Rochester, Minn.: Whiting Press, 1960.

Badian, N. "Auditory-Visual Integration, Auditory Memory, and Reading in Retarded and Adequate Readers. *Journal of Learning Disabilities* 10(1977):49–54.

Boucher, S. "The Effects of Memory Training on Reading Achievement." Master's thesis, California State University, Fresno, 1976.

Bryden, M. "Auditory-Visual and Sequential Spatial Matching in Relation to Reading Ability." *Child Development* 43(1972):824–32.

Carpenter, R. "Case Study of an Auditory Dyslexic." *Journal of Learning Disabilities* 5(1972):121–30.

Chall, J. *Learning to Read: The Great Debate.* New York: McGraw-Hill, 1967.

Downing, J. *The Initial Teaching Alphabet Reading Experiment.* Glenview, Ill.: Scott Foresman, 1965.

Durrell, D., and Murphy, M. "The Auditory Discrimination Factor in Reading Readiness and Reading Disability." *Journal of Education* 140(1958):556–60.

Ealck, V. "Auditory Processing for the Child with Language Disorders." *Exceptional Children* 39(1973):413–17.

Forrest, E. "The Visual-Auditory-Verbal Program." *Journal of Learning Disabilities* 5(1972):136–45.

Gardner, K. "The Initial Teaching Alphabet and the Remedial Reading Program." *The Australian Journal on Education of Backward Children,* December 1966, pp. 67–71.

Golden, N., and Steiner, S. "Auditory and Visual Functions in Good and Poor Readers." *Journal of Learning Disabilities* 2(1969):476–81.

Hammill, D., and Larsen, S. "The Relationship of Selected Auditory Perceptual Skills and Reading Ability." *Journal of Learning Disabilities* 7(1974):40–45.

Heilman, A. *Phonics in Proper Perspective.* Columbus, Ohio: Charles E. Merrill, 1964.

Kaliski, L. "Auditory-Vocal Activation: A Tool for Teaching Children with a Specific Language Disability." *Journal of Learning Disabilities* 10(1977):22–30.

Kaluger, G., and Kolson, C. *Reading and Learning Disabilities.* Columbus, Ohio: Charles E. Merrill, 1969.

Lane, A. "Severe Reading Disability and the Initial Teaching Alphabet." *Journal of Learning Disabilities* 7(1974):479–83.

Lindamood, P. "A Developmental Program of Auditory Perception and Reading Improvement." Master's thesis, University of Oregon, 1967.

Luria, A. *Higher Cortical Functions in Man.* New York: Basic Books, 1966.

Myklebust, H. *Auditory Disorders in Children.* New York: Grune and Stratton, 1954.

Orton, S. *Reading, Writing, and Speech Problems in Children.* 1937. Reprint. New York: W. W. Norton, 1964.

Price, D., and Price, J. "The Portland Blend System in Nottingham Readers: Don't Hide Between Covers." *CANHC-GRAM* 5(1977):3.

Rohr, A. *A Multi-District Use of Visual Training as an Instructional Approach in Elementary Education.* Duncan, Okla.: Optometric Extension Program Foundation, 1968.

Roswell, F., and Natchez, G., eds. *Reading Disability.* 3d rev. ed. New York: Basic Books, 1977.

Semel, E. "The Effects of Auditory Perceptual Training on the Performance of Second Graders on Tests of Auditory Perception." Doctoral dissertation, Boston University, 1972.

Serio, M., and Briggs, B. " An Auditory Approach to Phonics Instruction." *Academic Therapy Quarterly* 3(1967–68):123–30.

Spache, G. *Diagnosing and Correcting Reading Disabilities.* Boston: Allyn and Bacon, 1976a.

———. "A Summary of Apparently Successful Perceptual Training Programs." Table 16-2 in *Investigating the Issues in Reading Disabilities,* pp. 417–18. Boston: Allyn and Bacon, 1976b.

Spring, C. "Encoding Speed and Memory Span in Dyslexic Children." *Journal of Special Education* 10(1976):35–40.

Stern, C., ed. *We Discover Reading.* New York: Random House, 1976.

Tallal, P. "Auditory Perceptual Factors in Language and Learning Disabilities." In *The Neuropsychology of Learning Disorders,* edited by R. Knights and D. Bakker, pp. 315–25. Baltimore: University Park Press, 1976.

Traub, N., and Bloom, F. *Recipe for Reading.* Cambridge, Mass.: Educators Publishing Service, 1972.

Trela, T. *Fourteen Remedial Reading Methods.* Belmont, Calif.: Fearon Pitman, 1968.

Valett, R. *The Remediation of Learning Disabilities.* 2d ed. Belmont, Calif.: Fearon Pitman, 1974.

Venezky, R. "Prerequisites for Learning to Read." In *Cognitive Learning in Children,* edited by J. Levin and V. Allen, pp. 163–90. New York: Academic Press, 1976.

Wallach, G., and Goldsmith, S. "Language Based Learning Disabilities: Reading Is Language Too!" *Journal of Learning Disabilities* 10(1977):57–61.

Wiig, E., and Semel, E. "Comprehension of Linguistic Concepts Requiring Logical Operations." *Journal of Speech and Hearing Research* 16(1973):627–36.

———. *Language Disabilities in Children and Adolescents.* Columbus, Ohio: Charles E. Merrill, 1976.

Zedler, E. "Management of Reading in the Educational Program of Pupils with Neurologically Based Learning Problems." In *Reading Disability and Perception,* edited by G. Spache, pp. 103–12. Newark, Del.: International Reading Association, 1969.

Zovko, N. "Problems of Remediating Dyslexia and Dysgraphia." Unpublished paper, Center Suvag for Rehabilitation of Speech and Hearing, Zagreb, Yugoslavia, 1977.

Chapter Nine

Blanco, R. *Prescriptions for Children with Learning and Adjustment Problems.* Springfield, Ill.: Charles C. Thomas, 1972.

Campbell, D. "Typewriting Contrasted with Handwriting: A Circumvention Study of Learning Disabled Children." *Journal of Special Education* 7(1973):155–58.

Chall, J. *Learning to Read: The Great Debate.* New York: McGraw-Hill, 1967.

Connell, D. "Creative Writing before Reading." Napa, Calif.: Napa Valley Unified School District. Paper presented at the California Reading Association Conference, Anaheim, California, November 5, 1977.

Critchley, M. *The Dyslexic Child.* London: William Heinemann Medical Books, 1970.

Early, G., and Kephart, N. "Developing Perceptual-Motor Training and Academic Achievement." *Academic Therapy Quarterly* 4(1969):201–6.

Engelmann, S. *Preventing Failure in the Primary Grades.* New York: Simon and Schuster, 1969.

Fernald, G. *Remedial Techniques in Basic School Subjects.* New York: McGraw-Hill, 1943.

Frostig, M. "Education for Children with Learning Disabilities." In *Progress in Learning Disabilities,* vol. 1, edited by H. Myklebust. New York: Grune and Stratton, 1968.

Gillingham, A., and Stillman, B. *Remedial Training for Children with Specific Language Disability in Reading, Spelling, and Penmanship.* 7th ed. Cambridge, Mass.: Educators Publishing Service, 1965.

Hallahan, D., and Cruickshank, W. *Psychoeducational Foundations of Learning Disabilities.* Englewood Cliffs, N.J.: Prentice-Hall, 1973.

Halliwell, J., and Solan, H. "The Effects of a Supplemental Perceptual Training Program on Reading Achievement." *Exceptional Children* 38(1972):613–22.

Heckelman, R. "A Neurological Impress Method of Remedial Reading Instruction." *Academic Therapy Quarterly* 4(1969):277-82.

_____. *Solutions to Reading Problems.* San Rafael, Calif.: Academic Therapy Publications, 1976.

Itard, J. *The Wild Boy of Aveyron.* 1894. Reprint. New York: Appleton-Century-Crofts, 1962.

Ittelson, W., and Kilpatrick, F. "Experiments in Perception." *Scientific American* 185 (1951):50-55.

Jastak, J., and Jastak, S. *Wide Range Achievement Test Manual.* Wilmington, Del.: Guidance Associates, 1976.

Johnson, D. "Treatment Approaches to Dyslexia." In *Reading Disability and Perception,* edited by G. Spache, pp. 95-102. Newark, Del.: International Reading Association, 1969.

Jordan, D. *Dyslexia in the Classroom.* Columbus, Ohio: Charles E. Merrill, 1972.

Krippner, S. "Diagnostic and Remedial Use of the Minnesota Percepto-Diagnostic Test in a Reading Clinic." Paper presented at the annual meeting of the American Psychological Association, Chicago, Illinois, September 1965.

Luria, A. *Restoration of Function after Brain Injury.* New York: Macmillan/Pergamon, 1963.

McCormick, C., and Poetker, B. "Improvement in Reading Achievement through Perceptual-Motor Training." *Research Quarterly* 39(1968):627-33.

McCormick, C.; Schnobrich, J.; and Footlik, W. "The Effect of Perceptual-Motor Training on Reading Achievement." *Academic Therapy Quarterly* 14(1969):171-75.

McCoy, L. "Braille: A Language for Severe Dyslexics." *Journal of Learning Disabilities* 8(1975):26-32.

Orton, J. "The Orton-Gillingham Approach." In *The Disabled Reader: Education of the Dyslexic Child,* edited by J. Money, pp. 119-45. Baltimore: Johns Hopkins Press, 1966.

Porterfield, J. *A Multi-Sensory Sequential Reading Method.* San Rafael, Calif.: Academic Therapy Publications, 1976.

Seagoe, M. "Verbal Development in a Mongoloid." *Exceptional Children* 31(1965):269-76.

Slayback, C. "Writers Become Readers." *CANHC-GRAM* 9(1975):3.

Slingerland, B. *Training in Some Prerequisites for Beginning Reading.* Cambridge, Mass.: Educators Publishing Service, 1967.

_____. *Teacher's Manual: Screening Tests for Identifying Children with Specific Language Disability.* Cambridge, Mass.: Educators Publishing Service, 1969.

_____. *A Multi-Sensory Approach to Language Arts for Specific Language Disability Children: A Guide for Primary Teachers.* Cambridge, Mass.: Educators Publishing Service, 1971.

Spache, G. *Investigating the Issues of Reading Disabilities.* Boston: Allyn and Bacon, 1976.

Stuart, M. *Neurophysiological Insights into Teaching.* Palo Alto, Calif.: Pacific Books, 1963.

Tarnopol, L., and Tarnopol, M., eds. *Reading Disabilities: An International Perspective.* Baltimore: University Park Press, 1976.

Valett, R., and Valett, S. *Perceptual-Motor Transitions to Reading.* San Rafael, Calif.: Academic Therapy Publications, 1974.

Van den Honert, D. "A Neuropsychological Technique for Training Dyslexics." *Journal of Learning Disabilites* 10(1977):21-27.

Wilson, S.; Harris, C.; and Harris, M. "Effects of an Auditory Perceptual Remediation Program on Reading Performance." *Journal of Learning Disabilities* 9(1976):670-78.

Chapter Ten

Ackerman, P.; Peters, J.; and Dykman, R. "Children with Learning Disabilities: WISC

Profiles." *Journal of Learning Disabilities* 4(1971):150-66.

Alexandroff, M. *Hypnosis and Your Child.* St. Catharines, Ontario: Almost Diversified Publishing Co., 1972.

Ayres, A. *Sensory Integration and Learning Disorders.* Los Angeles: Western Psychological Services, 1972.

Barber, T. "The Necessary and Sufficient Conditions for Hypnotic Behavior." *American Journal of Clinical Hypnosis* 3(1960):31-42.

_____. "Physiological Effects of Hypnosis." *Psychological Bulletin* 58(1961):390-419.

Bender, N. "Self Verbalization versus Tutor Verbalization in Modifying Impulsivity." *Journal of Educational Psychology* 68(1976):347-54.

Bettelheim, B. *The Uses of Enchantment: The Meaning and Importance of Fairy Tales.* New York: Vintage Books, 1975.

Billingsley, F. "The Effects of Self and Externally Imposed Schedules of Reinforcement on Oral Reading Performance." *Journal of Learning Disabilities* 10(1977):549-50.

Bloomfield, H.; Cain, M.; Jaffe, D.; and Kory, R. *TM: Discovering Inner Energy and Overcoming Stress.* New York: Dell, 1975.

Brain/Mind Bulletin. *Report Card for the Other Side of the Brain.* P.O. Box 42211, Los Angeles, 1975.

Bronfenbrenner, U. "The Split Level American Family." In *The Formative Years,* edited by S. Coopersmith and R. Feldman, pp. 73-86. San Francisco: Albion Publishing Co., 1974.

Carr, R. *Creative Yoga Exercises for Children.* New York: Doubleday, 1973.

Carter, J., and Synolds, D. "Effects of Relaxation Training upon Handwriting Quality." *Journal of Learning Disabilities* 7(1974):274-83.

Clarke, L. *Can't Read, Can't Write, Can't Talk Too Good Either.* New York: Penguin Books, 1974.

Conners, C.; Rothschild, G.; Eisenberg, L.; Schwartz, L.; and Robinson, E. "Dextroamphetamine Sulfate in Children with Learn-

ing Disorders." *Archives of General Psychiatry* 21(1969):182-90.

Connor, J. *Classroom Activities for Helping Hyperactive Children.* New York: Center for Applied Research in Education, 1974.

Cott, A. "Megavitamins: The Orthomolecular Approach to Behavioral Disorders and Learning Disabilities." *Academic Therapy Quarterly* 7(1972):248.

Fagen, S.; Nicholas, J.; and Stevens, D. *Teaching Children Self-Control.* Columbus, Ohio: Charles E. Merrill, 1975.

Feingold, B. *Why Your Child Is Hyperactive.* New York: Random House, 1975.

Frank, J., and Levinson, H. "Dysmetric Dyslexia and Dyspraxia." *Academic Therapy Quarterly* 11(1975-76):133-42.

_____. "Anti-Motion Sickness Medications in Dysmetric Dyslexia and Dyspraxia." *Academic Therapy Quarterly* 12(1977):411-24.

Friedman, M.; Guyer-Christie, B.; and Tymchuk, A. "Cognitive Style and Specialized Hemispheric Processing in Learning Disability." In *The Neuropsychology of Learning Disorders,* edited by R. Knights and D. Bakker, pp. 257-63. Baltimore: University Park Press, 1976.

Gittelman-Klein, R. "Psychopharmacological Approaches to the Treatment of Learning Disability: Implications for Visual Processes." In *Basic Visual Processes and Learning Disabilities,* edited by G. Leisman. Springfield, Ill.: Charles C. Thomas, 1975.

Jampolsky, G. "Use of Hypnosis and Sensory Motor Stimulation to Aid Children with Learning Problems." *Journal of Learning Disabilities* 3(1970):29-34.

Journal of Learning Disabilities (Special Issue). "The Role of Medication in the Treatment of Learning Disabilities and Related Behavior Disorders." 4(1971):470-538.

Kiss, M. *Yoga for Young People.* New York: Bobbs-Merrill Co., 1971.

Krippner, S. "The Use of Hypnosis with Elementary and Secondary School Children in a Summer Reading Clinic." *American Journal of Clinical Hypnosis* 8(1966):261-66.

Lerer, R., and Lerer, M. "Response of Adolescents with Minimal Brain Dysfunction to Methylphenidate." *Journal of Learning Disabilities* 10(1977):35–40.

Levine, M. "Physiological Responses in Intrasensory and Intersensory Integration of Auditory and Visual Signals by Normal and Deficit Readers." In *The Neuropsychology of Learning Disorders,* edited by R. Knights and D. Bakker, pp. 99–110. Baltimore: University Park Press, 1976.

Linden, W. "Practicing of Meditation by School Children and Their Levels of Field Dependence-Independence, Test Anxiety, and Reading Achievement." *Journal of Consulting and Clinical Psychology* 41(1973): 139–43.

Lupin, M.; Braud, L.; Braud, W.; and Duer, W. "Children, Parents, and Relaxation Tapes." *Academic Therapy Quarterly* 12 (1976):105–13.

Luria, A. *The Working Brain: An Introduction to Neuropsychology.* New York: Basic Books, 1973.

McClelland, D.; Atkinson, J.; Clark, R.; and Lowell, E. *The Achievement Motive.* New York: Appleton-Century-Crofts, 1953.

McCord, H. "Hypnotherapy and Stuttering." *Journal of Clinical and Experimental Hypnosis* 3(1955):210–14.

McCormick, C., and Poetker, B. "Improvement in Reading Achievement through Perceptual-Motor Training." *Research Quarterly* 39(1968):627–33.

Meichenbaum, D. "Cognitive-Functional Approach to Cognitive Factors as Determinants of Learning Disabilities." In *The Neuropsychology of Learning Disorders,* edited by R. Knights and D. Bakker, pp. 423–41. Baltimore: University Park Press, 1976.

Moyer, S., and Newcomer, P. "Reversals in Reading: Diagnosis and Remediation." *Exceptional Children* 43(1977):424–30.

New York Times Western Edition. "Painless Learning." March 8, 1963.

Oettinger, L. "Medical versus Psychological Treatment of Attention Disorders in Boys."

Symposium presentation at the California State Psychological Association Convention, San Francisco, January 6, 1978.

Ornstein, R. *The Nature of Human Consciousness.* San Francisco: W. H. Freeman, 1973.

Park, G., and Schneider, K. "Thyroid Function in Relation to Dyslexia." *Journal of Reading Behavior* 7(1975):197–99.

Parker, W. *Prayer Can Change Your Life.* Englewood Cliffs, N.J.: Prentice-Hall, 1957.

Parry, P. "The Effect of Reward on the Performance of Hyperactive Children." Doctoral dissertation, McGill University, Montreal, 1973.

Pine, M. "Reading, Self-Concept, and Informal Education." In *Learner Centered Teaching,* edited by G. Pine and A. Boy, pp. 143–69. Denver: Love Publications, 1977.

Pribam, K., and McGuiness, D. "Activation and the Control of Attention." *Psychological Review* 82(1975):116–49.

Puharich, H. "Psychic Research and the Healing Process." In *Psychic Exploration: A Challenge for Science,* edited by E. Mitchell, pp. 333–47. New York: G. P. Putnam, 1974.

Radin, N. "The Impact of a Kindergarten Home Counseling Program." *Exceptional Children* 36(1969):251–56.

Rimland, B. "High-Dosage Levels of Certain Vitamins in the Treatment of Children with Severe Mental Disorder." In *Orthomolecular Psychiatry,* edited by D. Hawkins and L. Pauling, pp. 513–43. San Francisco: W. H. Freeman, 1973.

Sanders, D. "Study Panel Urges Increased Role for Arts in U.S. Schools." *Fresno Bee,* June 12, 1977.

Schaefer, C. "Motivation: A Major Cause of School Under-Achievement." *Devereuk Forum* 12(1977):16–29.

Scholastic Magazine. *Reading in the Home* (brochure). 50 West Forty-fourth Street, New York, undated.

The School Psychology Digest 5(1976):1–48.

Schpoont, S. "Hypnosis: Does It Have a Place in the Schools?" Paper presented at the

American Psychological Association Convention, Montreal, Canada, August 28, 1973.

Simpson, D., and Nelson, A. "Attention Training through Breathing Control to Modify Hyperactivity." *Journal of Learning Disabilities* 7(1974):274–83.

Smith, L. *Improving Your Child's Behavior Chemistry*. Englewood Cliffs, N.J.: Prentice-Hall, 1976.

Smith, M. "School and Home: Focus on Achievement." In *Developing Programs for the Educationally Disadvantaged*, edited by A. Passow, pp. 89–107. New York: Teachers College Press, 1968.

Staats, A., and Butterfield, W. "Treatment of Nonreading in a Culturally Deprived Juvenile Delinquent: An Application of Reinforcement Principles." *Child Development* 36(1965):925–42

Tarver, S.; Hallahan, D.; Kauffman, J.; and Ball, D. "Verbal Rehearsal and Selective Attention in Children with Learning Disabilities: A Developmental Lag." *Journal of Experimental Child Psychology* 22(1976): 375–78.

Valett, R. *The Practice of School Psychology*. New York: John Wiley, 1963.

_____. *Modifying Children's Behavior: A Guide for Parents and Professionals*. Belmont, Calif.: Fearon Pitman, 1969.

_____. *Effective Teaching: A Guide to Diagnostic Prescriptive Task Analysis*. Belmont, Calif.: Fearon Pitman, 1970.

_____. *The Psychoeducational Treatment of Hyperactive Children*. Belmont, Calif.: Fearon Pitman, 1974.

_____. "Human Behavior Modification." In *Humanistic Education: Developing the Total Person*, pp. 171–86. St. Louis: C. V. Mosby, 1977.

Walters, R., and Doan, H. "Perceptual and Cognitive Functioning of Retarded Readers." *Journal of Consulting Psychology* 26(1962):355–61.

Wender, P. "Hypothesis for a Possible Biochemical Basis of Minimal Cerebral Dysfunction." In *The Neuropsychology of Learning Disorders*, edited by R. Knights and D. Bakker. pp. 111–24. Baltimore: University Park Press, 1976.

Wilson, C. *New Pathways in Psychology*. London: Victor Gollanez, 1972.

Chapter Eleven

Algozzine, R., and Sutherland, J. "Non-Psychoeducational Foundations of Learning Disabilities." *Journal of Special Education* 11(1977):91–98.

Ashton-Warner, S. *Teacher*. New York: Simon and Schuster, 1963.

Bloom, B., and Krathwohl, D., eds. *Taxonomy of Educational Objectives: Handbook I: Cognitive Domain*. New York: Longmans, Green and Co., 1956.

Brueckner, L., and Bond, G. *The Diagnosis and Treatment of Learning Difficulties*. New York: Appleton-Century-Crofts, 1955.

Coleman, J. "Perceptual Retardation in Reading Disability Cases." *Journal of Educational Psychology* 44(1953):497–503.

Cratty, B. "Uses of Movement in Eliciting High Level Cognitive Activity in Children and Youth." Paper presented to the International Council of Sport and Physical Education sponsored by UNESCO, Eleventh Annual Meeting of the Research Committee, Rome, Italy, September 26–October 1, 1971a.

_____. *Active Learning: Games to Enhance Academic Abilities*. Englewood Cliffs, N.J.: Prentice-Hall, 1971b.

Cratty, B., and Martin, M. *The Effects of a Program of Learning Games Upon Selected Academic Abilities in Children with Learning Difficulties*. Washington, D.C.: Department of Health, Education and Welfare, Office of Education, Division of Handicapped Children, 1971.

Dale, P. *Language Development: Structure and Function*. Hinsdale, Ill.: Dryden Press, 1972.

Fishbein, J. "Reading and Linguistics." Reprinted from *The Instructor.* Chicago: Science Research Associates, 1967.

Garber, H. "The Milwaukee Project." Address to the International Seminar on the Education of Exceptional Children, Lund, Sweden, July 14, 1977.

Guilford, J. *The Nature of Human Intelligence.* New York: McGraw-Hill, 1967.

Heber, R.; Garber, H.; Harrington, S.; Hoffman, C.; and Falender, C. "Rehabilitation of Families at Risk for Mental Retardation: Progress Report." Madison, Wis.: University of Wisconsin, Rehabilitation Research and Training Center in Mental Retardation, 1972.

Inhelder, B., and Piaget, J. *The Growth of Logical Thinking from Childhood to Adolescence.* New York: Basic Books, 1958.

Patton, P. "Beyond Sesame Street," *United Air Lines Mainliner,* October 1977, pp. 52-56.

Reitan, R. "Certain Differential Effects of Left and Right Cerebral Lesions in Human Adults." *Journal of Comparative and Physiological Psychology* 48(1955):474-77.

Rich, A., and Nedboy, R. "Hey Man We're Writing a Poem." *Teaching Exceptional Children* 9(1977):92-94.

Robinson, R. *An Introduction to the Cloze Procedure.* Newark, Del.: International Reading Association, 1971.

Roswell, F., and Natchez, G., eds. *Reading Disability.* New York: Basic Books, 1977.

Rowen, B. *Learning through Movement.* New York: Teachers College Press, Columbia University, 1963.

Skinner, B. F. "The Technology of Teaching." *Proceedings of the Royal Society* 162 (1965):427-43.

Smith, L.; Adams, R.; Schomer, J.; and Willardson, M. "Skills through Self-Recording." *Today's Education.* NEW Journal, January 1971, pp. 19-20.

Spector, R. "Neuropsychological Approach to the Diagnosis and Remediation of Reading Disability (Dyslexia)." Paper presented at the California State Psychological Association Convention, San Francisco, January 7, 1978.

Strang, R. "Step by Step Instruction in Beginning Reading for Slow Learners." *Exceptional Children* 31(1965):31-36.

Vaille, L. "Educational Approach to Dyslexia." *CANHC-GRAM* 9(1975):1-2.

Valett, R. *Developing Cognitive Abilities: Teaching Children to Think.* St. Louis: C. V. Mosby, 1978.

Vogel, S. *Syntactic Disabilities in Normal and Dyslexic Children.* Baltimore: University Park Press, 1975.

_____. "Morphological Ability in Normal and Dyslexic Children." *Journal of Learning Disabilities* 10(1977):41-49.

Walters, R., and Doan, H. "Perceptual and Cognitive Functioning of Retarded Readers," *Journal of Consulting Psychology* 26(1962):355-61.

Wiig, E., and Semel, E. *Language Disabilities in Children and Adolescents.* Columbus, Ohio: Charles E. Merrill, 1976.

Wilson, R. *Diagnostic and Remedial Reading for Classroom and Clinic.* 2d ed. Columbus, Ohio: Charles E. Merrill, 1972.

Chapter Twelve

Christensen, A. *Luria's Neuropsycholgical Investigation.* New York: John Wiley/Spectrum, 1975.

Dolch, E. *Teaching Primary Reading,* Champaign, Ill.: Garrard Publishing Company, 1960.

Halstead, W. *Brain and Intelligence: A Quantitative Study of the Frontal Lobes.* Chicago: University of Chicago Press, 1947.

Luria A. *Basic Problems in Neurolinguistics.* The Hague, Netherlands: Mouton, 1976.

Luria, A., and Majovski, L. "Basic Approaches Used in American and Soviet Clinical Neuropsychology." *American Psychologist* 32 (1977):959-68.

Reitan, R., and Davidson, L. *Clinical Neuropsychology Current Status and Applications.* New York: Winston-Wiley, 1974.

Thomas, G., and Cresimbeni, J. *Guiding the Gifted Child.* New York: Random House, 1966.

Chapter Thirteen

Anderson, I.; Hughes, B.; and Dixon, W. "Age of Learning to Read and Its Relation to Sex, Intelligence, and Reading Achievement in the Sixth Grade." *Journal of Educational Research* 49(1956):447-53.

Axelrod, S. *Behavior Modification for the Classroom Teacher.* New York: McGraw-Hill, 1977.

Bakker, D.; Teunissen, J.; and Bosch, J. "Development of Laterality-Reading Patterns." In *The Neuropsychology of Learning Disorders,* edited by R. Knights and D. Bakker, pp. 207-20. Baltimore: University Park Press, 1976.

Bakker, D., and Van Rijnsoever, R. *Language Proficiency and Lateral Position in the Classroom.* Towson, Md.: The Orton Society, 1977.

Bell, A.; Abrahamson, D.; and McRae, K. "Reading Retardation: A 12 Year Prospective Study." *Journal of Pediatrics* 91(1977): 363-70.

Belmont, L., and Birch, H. "Lateral Dominance, Lateral Awareness, and Reading Disabilities." *Child Development* 38(1967):827-33.

Bennett, N. *Teaching Styles and Pupil Progress.* London: Open Books, 1976.

Bettelheim, B. *The Children of the Dream.* New York: Macmillan, 1969.

Blau, T. "Torque and Schizophrenic Vulnerability." *American Psychologist* 32(1977): 997-1005.

Block, N., and Dworkin, G., eds. *The IQ Controversy.* New York: Pantheon, 1976.

Bloom, B. *Human Characteristics and School Learning.* New York: McGraw-Hill, 1976.

Bogan, J. "Some Educational Aspects of Hemispheric Specialization." *UCLA Educator* 17 (1975):24-32.

Bronfenbrenner, U. "The Psychological Costs of Quality and Equality in Education." *Child Development* 38(1967):909-25.

Buffery, A. "Sex Differences in the Neuropsychological Development of Verbs and Spatial Skills." In *The Neuropsychology of Learning Disorders,* edited by R. Knights and D. Bakker, pp. 187-206. Baltimore: University Park Press, 1976.

Cascario, E. "The Male Teacher and Reading Achievement of First Grade Boys and Girls." Doctoral dissertation, Lehigh University, 1972.

Croxen, M., and Lytton, H. "Reading Disability and Difficulties in Finger Localization and Right-Left Discrimination." *Developmental Psychology* 5(1971):256-62.

Denckla, M. "The Neurological Basis of Reading Disability." In *Reading Disability,* 3d rev. ed., edited by F. Roswell and G. Natchez. New York: Basic Books, 1977.

Dykstra, R., and Tinney, R. "Sex Differences in Reading Readiness: First Grade Achievement and Second Grade Achievement." In *Reading and Realism,* edited by J. Figurel, pp. 623-28. Newark, Del.: International Reading Association, 1969.

Erman, R. "Elementary Children's Preferences for Ethnicity and Sex of Teachers." Doctoral dissertation, University of Southern California, 1973.

Eysenck, H. J. *The Inequality of Man.* San Diego: Edits Publishers, 1975.

Feingold, B. "It's a Shame He Just Can't Read." Eyewitness News, videotape. Oakland, Calif., 1973.

Gates, A. "Sex Differences in Reading Ability." *Elementary School Journal* 61(1961):431-34.

Gentile, A. *Further Studies in Achievement Testing of Hearing Impaired Students.* United States: Spring 1971, series D, number 13. Annual Survey of Hearing Impaired Children and Youth. Washington, D.C.: Gallaudet College, Office of Demographic Studies, 1973.

Gesell, A. *The First Five Years of Life: A Guide*

to the *Study of the Pre-School Child.* New York: Harper & Row, 1940.

Herron, J. "South Paws: How Are They Different?" *Psychology Today,* March 1976, pp. 50–56.

Hirst, W. "Sex as a Predictor Variable for Success in First Grade Reading Achievement." *Journal of Learning Disabilities* 2(1969):23–28.

Hughes, M. "Sex Differences in Reading Achievement in the Elementary Grades." *Supplementary Educational Monographs* 77 (1953):102–6.

Ilg, F., and Ames, L. *School Readiness.* New York: Harper & Row, 1965.

Jastak, J., and Jastak, S. *Wide Range Achievement Test Manual.* Wilmington, Del.: Guidance Associates, 1976.

Jensen, A. "How Much Can We Boost IQ and Scholastic Achievement?" *Harvard Educational Review* 39(1969):1–123.

Kagan, J. "Acquisition and Significance of Sex Typing and Sex Role Identity." In *Review of Child Development Research,* vol. 1, edited by M. Hoffman and L. Hoffman, pp. 137–68. New York: Russell Sage Foundation, 1964.

Kernkamp, E., and Price, E. "Coeducation May Be A 'No-No' for the Six-Year-Old Boy." *Phi Delta Kappan* 53(1972):662–63.

Konski, V. "An Investigation into Differences between Boys and Girls in Selected Reading Readiness Areas and in Reading Achievement." Doctoral dissertation, University of Missouri, 1951.

Light, H. *Light's Retention Scale.* San Rafael, Calif.: Academic Therapy Publications, 1977.

Lyles, T. "Grouping by Sex." *National Elementary School Principal* 46(1966):38–41.

Maccoby, E., and Jacklin, C. "Myth, Reality and Shades of Gray: What We Know and Don't Know about Sex Differences." *Psychology Today,* December 1974, pp. 109–12.

Mead, M. *Male and Female.* New York: William Morrow and Co., 1949.

Montgomery, M. *POINT.* Fresno, Calif.: Fresno Unified School District, 1971.

Rader, D. "Against Coeducation." *Playboy,* January 1977, pp. 40–41.

Samuels, F. "Sex Differences in Reading Achievement." *Journal of Educational Research* 36(1943):594–603.

Smith, F. "Making Sense of Reading and of Reading Instruction." *Harvard Educational Review* 47(1977):386–95.

Smith, L. *Improving Your Child's Behavior Chemistry.* Englewood Cliffs, N.J.: Prentice-Hall, 1976.

Stanchfield, J. "Development of Prereading Skills in an Experimental Kindergarten Program." *Reading Teacher* 24(1971):699–707.

Tregaskis, E. "The Relationship Between Sex Role Standards of Reading and Reading Achievement of First Grade Boys." Doctoral dissertation, State University of New York, Albany, 1972.

Trotter, R. "Sinister Psychology." *Science News* 106(1974):220–22.

Valett, R. *The Practice of School Psychology.* New York: John Wiley, 1963.

_____. *Developing Cognitive Abilities: Teaching Children to Think.* St. Louis: C. V. Mosby, 1978.

Vellutino, F. "Alternative Conceptualization of Dyslexia: Evidence in Support of a Verbal-Deficit Hypothesis." *Harvard Educational Review* 47(1977):334–49.

Wechsler, D. *The Measurement of Adult Intelligence.* 3d ed. Baltimore: Williams and Wilkins Co., 1988.

Chapter Fourteen

Bakker, D. *Hemispheric Specialization and Stages in the Learning to Read Process.* Towson, Md.: The Orton Society, 1973.

Danenhower, H. *Teaching Adults with Specific Language Disability.* Towson, Md.: The Orton Society, 1972.

Duane, D., and Rawson, M., eds. *Reading,*

Perception, and Language. Baltimore: New York Press, 1974.

Gillingham, A. "Detailed Description of Remedial Work for Reading, Spelling, and Penmanship." In *Education and Specific Language Disability: The Papers of Anna Gillingham,* edited by S. Childs, pp. 111-50. Towson, Md.: The Orton Society, 1968.

Hallahan, D.; Gajar, A.; Cohen, S.; and Tarver, S. "Selective Attention and Locus of Control in Learning Disabled and Normal Children." *Journal of Learning Disabilities* 11(1978):231-36.

Karnes, L. *Dyslexia in Special Education.* Towson, Md.: The Orton Society, 1964.

Kaszniak, A. "Dichotic Auditory Vigilance during Feedback-Enhanced EEG Alpha." *Psychophysiology* 10(1973):203.

Oliver, M. "Looking at Word Pictures." *Reading Teacher* 22(1969):426-29.

O'Malley, J., and Comers, C. "The Effect of Unilateral Alpha Training on Visual-Evoked Response in a Dyslexic Adolescent." *Psychophysiology* 9(1972):467.

Orton, S. "World-Blindness in School Children." *Archives of Neurology and Psychiatry* 14(1925):581-615.

_____. *Reading, Writing, and Speech Problems in Children.* 1937. Reprint. New York: W. W. Norton, 1964.

Robbins, A., and Sibley, L. *Creative Art Therapy.* New York: Brunner-Mazel, 1976.

Satterfield, J., and Dawson, M. "Electrodermal Correlates of Hyperactivity in Children." *Psychophysiology* 8(1971):191.

Tomatis, A. *Éducation et Dyslexie.* Collection science de l'education. Les Éditions ESF, Paris, 1972.

Valett, R. *The Psychoeducational Treatment of Hyperactive Children.* Belmont, Calif.: Fearon Pitman, 1974.

_____. *Developing Cognitive Abilities: Teaching Children to Think.* St. Louis: C. V. Mosby, 1978.

Wolf, C. *Experimental Investigation of Specific Language Disability (Dyslexia).* Towson, Md.: The Orton Society, 1967.

Materials

Active Learning—Games to Enhance Academic Abilities, Prentice-Hall Media

Auditory Discrimination in Depth Program (ADD), Teaching Resources Corporation

Auditory Perception Training Program, Developmental Learning Materials

Basic Reading Series, Science Research Associates, Inc.

Bender Gestalt Test for Children, Charles E. Merrill Publishing Company

Bender-Purdue Reflex Test and Training Manual, Academic Therapy Publications

BFA Comprehension Skill Laboratory, BFA Educational Media

Binaural Auditory Trainers, AMBCO Electronics

Boehm Test of Verbal Concepts, Psychological Corporation

California Achievement Test, CTB/McGraw-Hill Division

California Reading Test, *see* California Achievement Test

California Test of Mental Maturity—Primary Series CTB/McGraw-Hill Division

Comp IV, Milton Bradley Company

Comprehensive Test of Basic Skills—Level A, CTB/McGraw-Hill Division

Critical Thinking Program, Midwest Publications Company, Inc.

Design Sequence Cards, Academic Therapy Publications

Detroit Tests of Learning Aptitude, Bobbs-Merrill Company, Inc.

Developing Auditory Awareness and Insight, Instructional Materials and Equipment Distributors

Developing Learning Readiness, Webster Division, McGraw-Hill Book Company

Developing Reading Skills, Educational Enrichment Materials

Developing Visual Awareness and Insight, Instructional Materials and Equipment Distributors

Developmental Syntax Program, Learning Concepts, Inc.

DISTAR Program, Science Research Associates, Inc.

Dolch Basic Sight Word Materials, Garrard Publishing Company

Dr. Seuss Beginning Readers, Random House

Durrell Analysis of Reading Difficulty, Harcourt Brace Jovanovich, Inc.

Edmark Reading Program, Edmark Associates

Electro-Tach, Lafayette Instrument Company

EP Basic Reading Program, Educational Projections Company

ETA Electronics Reading System, Educational Teaching Aids

Fables of Aesop, Prentice-Hall Media

First Thinking Box I, Benefic Press

Fitzhugh Plus Program, Allied Education Council

Form-A-Phrase Board, Scitronics, Inc.

Franzblau Multi-Sensory Coordinator, Keystone View Company

Friendly Tutor, Creative Teaching Associates

Frostig Developmental Test of Visual Perception, Consulting Psychologists Press, Inc.

Frostig Program for the Development of Visual Perception, Follett Publishing Company

Functional Word Recognition, Mast Development Company

Fun with Phonics, Highlights for Children, Inc.

Galaxy 5 Series, Fearon Pitman Publishers, Inc.

Gates-MacGinitie Reading Tests, Teachers College Press, Columbia University

Gilmore Oral Reading Test, Harcourt Brace Jovanovich, Inc.

The Goldman-Fristoe-Woodcock Auditory Skills Test Battery, American Guidance Service

GOAL Language Development Program, Milton Bradley Company

Goodenough Draw-A-Person Test: Measurement of Intelligence by Drawings, Harcourt Brace Jovanovich, Inc.

Gray Oral Reading Test, Bobbs-Merrill Company

Halstead Aphasia Screening Test, Industrial Relations Center, University of Chicago

Halstead-Reitan Neuropsychological Test Battery, Ralph Reitan Neuropsychological Laboratory

Handtalk, Childcraft Education Corporation

Harris Tests of Lateral Dominance, Psychological Corporation

Hooper Visual Organization Test, Western Psychological Services

Hyperactive Rating Scales, Fearon Pitman Publishers, Inc.

Illinois Test of Psycholinguistic Abilities (ITPA), University of Illinois Press

Initial Teaching Alphabet Publications (i.t.a.), Fearon Pitman Publishers, Inc.

Innerchange, Pennant Educational Materials

Iowa Every Pupil Test, see Iowa Tests of Basic Skills

Iowa Tests of Basic Skills, Houghton Mifflin Company

Johnny Right-to-Read Program, Academic Therapy Publications

Jordon Left-Right Reversal Test, Academic Therapy Publications

Keystone Integrator, Keystone View Company

Kinesthetic Alphabet, R. H. Stone Products

Language Structure Simplified, Educational Activities, Inc.

Language-Structured Auditory Retention Span Test, Academic Therapy Publications

Larsen-Hammill Test of Written Spelling, Academic Therapy Publications

Learning Language at Home, Council for Exceptional Children

Learning with Laughter, Prentice-Hall Media

Lee-Clark Reading Readiness Test, CTB/McGraw-Hill Division

Leir Language Experience in Reading Program, Encyclopaedia Britannica Educational Corporation

Leiter International Performance Scale, C. H. Stoelting Company

Lindamood Auditory Conceptualization Test, Teaching Resources Corporation

Lorge-Thorndike Intelligence Tests, Houghton Mifflin Company

LSI Reading Skills Development, Learning Skills, Inc.

Merlin, Parker Brothers

The Metropolitan Achievement Test—Primary I, Harcourt Brace Jovanovich, Inc.

The Michigan Tracking Program, Ann Arbor Publishers

Minnesota Multiphasic Personality Inventory (MMPI), Psychological Corporation

NFL Reading Kit, Bowmar Publishing Corporation

Pacemaker Bestellers, Fearon Pitman Publishers, Inc.

Peabody Language Development Kits, American Guidance Service, Inc.

Peabody Picture Vocabulary Test (PPVT), American Guidance Service, Inc.

Peabody Rebus Reading Program, American Guidance Service, Inc.

Peace, Harmony, and Awareness Self-Management Tapes, Melton Book Company, Inc.

The Pelican Series, Allyn and Bacon, Inc.

Perceive and Respond Auditory Program, Modern Education Corporation

Perceptualmotor Pen, Wayne Engineering

Perceptual Skills Curriculum, Walker Educational Book Corporation

Phonic Mirror, H.C. Electronics, Inc.

Phonics We Use Games, Lyons and Carnahan

PIPER, Reader's Digest Services, Inc.

Productive Thinking Program, Charles E. Merrill Publishing Company

Psychoeducational Inventory of Basic Learning Abilities, Fearon Pitman Publishers, Inc.

Quick Neurological Screening Test, Academic Therapy Publications

RADEA, Melton Book Company

Reading Laboratory Series, Science Research Associates, Inc.

Reading-Thinking Skills, Continental Press, Inc.

Reading via Typing, AVKO

Rebus Reading Programs, American Guidance Service, Inc.

Recipe for Reading, Educators Publishing Services, Inc.

REC Talking Page, Response Environments Corporation

Remedial Training for Children with Specific Disability in Reading, Spelling and Penmanship, Educators Publishing Services, Inc.

Rhyming—Levels A, B, C, Continental Press, Inc.

Santa Clara Plus, Richard L. Zweig Associates

Screening Test for Auditory Perception, Academic Therapy Publications

Seashore Measures of Musical Talents, Psychological Corporation

Semel Auditory Processing Programs, Follett Publishing Company

Simon, Milton Bradley Company

Skill Builder, Reader's Digest Services, Inc.

Skyline Series, Webster Division, McGraw-Hill Book Company

Slingerland Tests of Specific Language Disability, Educators Publishing Service, Inc.

SOBAR Criterion Tests, Science Research, Associates, Inc.

Southern California Sensory Integration Tests, Western Psychological Services

Spache Diagnostic Reading Scales, CTB/McGraw-Hill Division

Spatial Organization Workbooks I, II, III (Fitzhugh Plus Program), Allied Education Council

Special Language Audio Flashcard Program, Electronic Futures, Inc.

Specter Series, Fearon Pitman Publishers, Inc.

SRA Corrective Reading Program, Science Research Associates, Inc.

Stanford Achievement Test, Harcourt Brace Jovanovich, Inc.

Stanford Diagnostic Reading Test—Level 1, Harcourt Brace Jovanovich, Inc.

STEP Language Board and Language Strips, L.A. Hatch Company

Structural Reading Series, L.W. Singer Company

Sullivan Programmed Reading, Webster Division, McGraw-Hill Book Company

Syntax One, Communication Skill Builders, Inc.

System 80, Borg-Wagner Educational Systems

Tales of Fantasy and Music, Prentice-Hall Media

3-D Test for Visualization Skill, Academic Therapy Publications

Thinking Skills Development Program II, Benefic Press

Think Language Program, Innovative Science, Inc.

Tutorgram, Enrichment Reading Corporation of America

Valett Developmental Survey of Basic Learning Abilities, Consulting Psychologists Press

Valett Perceptual-Motor Transitions to Reading Program, Academic Therapy Publications

Visual Discrimination, Continental Press, Inc.

Visual Echo II, Visual Echo Company

Visual Language Materials, Newby Visual Language, Inc.

Visual Perceptual Skills Filmstrips, Educational Records Sales

Visual Readiness Skills, Continental Press, Inc.

Visual Word Perception Cards, Academic Therapy Publications

The Wechsler Intelligence Scale for Children (WISC), Psychological Corporation

Wepman Auditory Discrimination Test, Joseph Wepman

Wide Range Achievement Tests (WRAT), Guidance Associates of Delaware, Inc.

Wide Range Reading and Spelling Test, Guidance Associates of Delaware, Inc.

Woodcock Reading Mastery Tests for Word Identification and Word Attack, American Guidance Service, Inc.

Zweig-Bruno Stereo-Tracing Exercise Program, Keystone View Company

Sources

Academic Therapy Publications, 1539 Fourth Street, San Rafael, Calif. 94901

Allied Education Council, Distribution Center, Galien, Mich. 49113

Allyn and Bacon, Inc., Longwood Division, Link Drive, Rockleigh, N.J. 07647

AMBCO Electronics, 1224 West Washington Boulevard, Los Angeles, Calif. 90007

American Guidance Service, Inc., Publishers' Building, Circle Pines, Minn. 55014

Ann Arbor Publishers, 610 South Forest, Ann Arbor, Mich. 48404

AVKO, 3084 West Willard Road, Birch Run, Mich. 48415

Benefic Press, 10300 West Roosevelt Road, Westchester, Ill. 60153

BFA Educational Media, P.O. Box 1795, Santa Monica, Calif. 90406

Biofeedback Research Institute, 6233 Wilshire Boulevard, Los Angeles, Calif. 90048

Bobbs-Merrill Co., Inc., 4300 West Sixty-second Street, Indianapolis, Ind. 46208

Borg-Wagner Educational Systems, 600 West University Drive, Arlington Heights, Ill. 60004

Bowmar Publishing Corporation, 4563 Colorado Boulevard, Los Angeles, Calif. 90039

Childcraft Education Corporation, 20 Kilmer Road, Edison, N.J. 08817

Child Guidance Toys, New York, N.Y.

Communication Skill Builders, Inc., 817 East Broadway, P.O. Box 6081-C, Tucson, Ariz. 85733

Consulting Psychologists Press, Inc., 577 College Avenue, Palo Alto, Calif. 94306

Continental Press, Inc., Elizabethtown, Pa. 17002

Council for Exceptional Children, Publications Sales, 1920 Association Drive, Reston, VA. 22091

Creative Teaching Associates, P.O. Box 7714, Fresno, Calif. 93727

CTB/McGraw-Hill Division, Del Monte Research Park, Monterey, Calif. 93940

Developmental Learning Materials, 7440 Natchez Avenue, Niles, Ill. 60648

Edmark Associates, 13241 Northup Way, Bellevue, Wash. 98005

Educational Activities, Inc., P.O. Box 392, Freeport, N.Y. 11520

Educational Enrichment Materials, Feik-Vaughn Associates, 145 Stuyvesant Drive, San Anselmo, Calif. 94960

Educational Projections Company, 3070 Lake Terrace, Glenview, Ill. 60025

Educational Records Sales, 157 Chambers Street, New York, N.Y. 10021

Educational Teaching Aids, A. Daigger and Company, 159 West Kinzie Street, Chicago, Ill. 60610

Educators Publishing Service, Inc., 75 Moulton Street, Cambridge, Mass. 02138

Electronic Futures, Inc., 57 Dodge Avenue, North Haven, Conn. 06473

Encyclopaedia Britannica Educational Corporation, 425 North Michigan Avenue, Chicago, Ill. 60611

Enrichment Reading Corporation of America, Iron Ridge, Wisc. 53035

Fearon Pitman Publishers, Inc., 6 Davis Drive, Belmont, Calif. 94002

Follett Publishing Company, 1010 West Washington Boulevard, Chicago, Ill. 60607

Garrard Publishing Company, 1607 North Market Street, Champaign, Ill. 61820

Guidance Associates of Delaware, Inc., 1526 Gilpin Avenue, Wilmington, Del. 19806

Harcourt Brace Jovanovich, Inc., 757 Third Avenue, New York, N.Y. 10017

L. A. Hatch Company, 24230 Mariano Street, Woodland Hills, Calif. 91367

H. C. Electronics, Inc., 250 Camino Alto, Mill Valley, Calif. 94941

Highlights for Children, Inc., 2300 West Fifth Avenue, Columbus, Ohio 43216

Houghton Mifflin Co., Test Department, P.O. Box 1970, Iowa City, Iowa 52240

Industrial Relations Center, University of Chicago, 1225 East Sixtieth Street, Chicago, Ill. 60637

Innovative Science, Inc., 300 Broad Street, Stamford, Conn. 06901

Instructional Materials and Equipment Distributors, 1415 Westwood Boulevard, Los Angeles, Calif. 90024

Keystone View Company, Meadville, Pa. 16335

Lafayette Instrument Company, P.O. Box 1279, Sagamore Parkway, LaFayette, Ind. 47902

Learning Concepts, Inc., 2501 North Lamar, Austin, Texas 78705

Learning Skills, Inc., 900 Fullbright Avenue, Chatsworth, Calif. 91311

Lyons and Carnahan, 407 East Twenty-fifth Street, Chicago, Ill. 60610

Mast Development Company, 2212 East Twelfth Street, Davenport, Iowa 52803

Melton Book Company, Inc., 111 Leslie Street, Dallas, Tex. 75207

Charles E. Merrill Publishing Co., 1300 Alum Creek Drive, Columbus, Ohio 43216

Midwest Publications Co., Inc., P.O. Box 129, Troy, Mich. 48099

Milton Bradley Company, 74 Park Street, Springfield, Mass. 01105

Modern Education Corporation, P.O. Box 721, Tulsa, Okla. 74101

Newby Visual Language, Inc., P.O. Box 121 AEN, Eagleville, Pa. 19408

Parker Brothers, P.O. Box 1006, Beverly, Mass. 01915

Pennant Educational Materials, 8265 Commercial Street, Suite 14-B, La Mesa, Calif. 92041

Prentice-Hall Media, Service Code HA2, 150 White Plains Road, Tarrytown, N.Y. 10591

Psychological Corporation, 757 Third Avenue, New York, N.Y. 10017

Random House, Westminster Distribution Center, 457 Hahn Road, Westminster, Md. 21157

Reader's Digest Services, Inc., Educational Division of Reader's Digest Association, Pleasantville, N.Y. 10570

Ralph Reitan Neuropsychological Laboratory, 1925 Thirty-eighth Avenue East, Seattle, Wash. 98112

Response Environments Corporation, 200 Silvan Avenue, Englewood Cliffs, N.J. 07632

Science Research Associates, Inc., 259 East Erie Street, Chicago, Ill. 60611

Scitronics, Inc., P.O. Box 5344, Bethlehem, Pa. 18015

L.W. Singer Company, 33 West Sixth Street, New York, N.Y. 10003

C.H. Stoelting Company, 1350 South Kostner Avenue, Chicago, Ill. 60623

R.H. Stone Products, P.O. Box 414, Detroit, Mich. 48232

Teachers College Press, Teachers College, Columbia University, 1234 Amsterdam Avenue, New York, N.Y. 10027

Teaching Resources Corporation, 100 Boylston Street, Boston, Mass. 02116

University of Illinois Press, 52 East Gregory Drive, Urbana, Ill. 61801

Visual Echo Company, 4 Godwin Avenue, Fair Lawn, N.J. 07410

Walker Educational Book Corporation, 720 Fifth Avenue, New York, N.Y. 10019

Wayne Engineering, Orthoptic Division, 4120 Greenwood, Skokie, Ill. 60076

Webster Division, McGraw-Hill Book Company, Book and Education Services Group, 1221 Avenue of the Americas, New York, N.Y. 10020

Joseph Wepman, 950 East Fifty-ninth Street, Chicago, Ill. 60637

Western Psychological Services, 12031 Wilshire Boulevard, Los Angeles, Calif. 90025

Richard L. Zweig Associates, 20800 Beach Boulevard, Huntington Beach, Calif. 92648

Index

Acetylcholine, role in neural growth, 36

Ackerman, Peters, and Dykman,1971, 25, 186

Active involvement, aid in developing reading comprehension, 222–224

Administrators, school, role in remedial language treatment, 53

Adult reading materials, 244–245
Materials: Galaxy 5, 245
Handtalk, 244
Innerchange, 244–245
Language Structure Simplified, 244
Pacemaker Bestellers, 244
The Productive Thinking Program, 244
Specter, 245

Age placement in school, as cause of learning problems, 12–13, 39, 247, 255

Alexandroff, 1972, 188

Alexia, description, 51
school remedial programs to treat, 53–57
team members to treat, 51–53

Algozzine and Sutherland, 1977, 214

Alpha training, 275

Altman and Dos, 1966, 36

Amblyopia, cause and treatment, 20

American Academy of Ophthalmology and Otolaryngology, 1960, 138

Ames, 1968, 12

Ammon and Ammon, 1971, 55

Amphetamines, use to increase cortical arousal, 13

Analysis, required in reading, 28

Anderson, Hughes, and Dixon, 1956, 248

Angular gyrus, maldevelopment, as cause of dyslexia, 79

Antivert. *See* Motion sickness medication

Anxiety, reducing, 82, 186–196
Lessons: Progressive Relaxation, 190–191
Relaxation through Self-Suggestion, 192–196

Aphasia, description, 50
school remedial programs to treat, 53–57
team members to treat, 51–53

Architecture, school, for handicapped, 256

Arena, 1968, 57

Arnold, Huestis, Wemmer, and Smeltzer, 1978, 57

Art activities, use in treatment, 275–276

Ashton-Warner, 1963, 215

Attention and motivation in reading, increasing, 186–211
anxiety reduction, 186–196
behavioral programming, 199, 202–206
nutrition and drug management, 207–209
parent support, 209–211
reinforcement, 197–199, 200–201

Auditory cortex, effect of dysfunction on phonetic analysis, 149

Auditory decoding, importance and remediation of, 142–144, 145–147
Lessons: Associating Words and Symbols, 146
Sound Symbol Discrimination, 145
Symbol Decoding, 147
Materials: The Auditory Discrimination in Depth Program, 143
Developing Auditory Awareness and Insight, 144

Semel Auditory Processing Programs, 144

Auditory dyslexia, 7

Auditory memory, importance and remediation of, 144, 148–149, 150–152
auditory-vocal activation, use, 148
Initial Teaching Alphabet, use, 144–145
Suvag Lingue, use, 148
Lessons: Basic Letter-Sound Associations, 151–152
Remembering Sequential Information, 150
Materials: Auditory Perception Training Programs, 148
Initial Teaching Alphabet Reading Program, 148
Special Language Audio Flashcard Program, 149

Auditory processing deficiencies, remediating, 137–160
auditory-vocal synthesis, 149, 153–159
decoding, 142–144, 145–147
dyslexic vs. nondyslexic, 16–20
importance of, 137–138
memory, 144, 148–149, 150–152
reception, 138–141

Auditory reception, importance and remediation of, 138–141
Lessons: Receptivity Training, 140
Rhyming, 141
Materials: Binaural Auditory Trainers, 139
Phonic Mirror, 139
Rhyming—Levels A, B, C, 139
Visual Echo II, 139

Auditory-visual integration, dyslexic vs. nondyslexic, 24–26